and **my allergies**
helped me coordinate my diet. . . .
—*A.S.*

The main thing I've noticed
since coming here is that I have *much* **more energy.**
Also, my eyes definitely look better, and I've lost
weight. I used to be very lethargic in the mornings and
now I actually get up earlier and with more energy. . .
.
—*C.V.*

Dr. Koyfman can guide you
through the process of cleansing the liver, gall
bladder, colon, small intestines, and stomach.
Everyone I know who has gone to him feels **happier,
healthier, and thinner, and is clearly much more
bright and energetic.**
—*D.G.*

**Find more
testimonials between the chapters and near the
end of the book.**

Healing through Cleansing

Book 2: Heal and Prevent

Sinus Problems

Tooth Decay

Ear Infection

Thyroid Dysfunction

Allergies

by Dr. Yakov Koyfman, N.D.

Practical Guide to a Healthy Lifestyle

Dedication

This little book is dedicated to the idea

That cleansing one's body of the toxins we take in
(from our food, water and air)
is an essential pathway to optimum health,

That natural techniques
which are gentle and powerfully effective
can and do remove the majority of these toxins,
and

That properly practicing
simple everyday cleansing procedures
is an important element
in one's overall detoxification program.

Cleansing procedures recommended in this book, may be used not only as prevention of disorders in the head organs, but also as an emergency help for soar throat, toothache, headache, sinuses, allergies, etc.

In order for these methods to work faster, it is important to catch the problem at the root, when first symptoms or pain are noticed. By doing so, you will not allow a light starting discomfort grow into a serious illness.

In This Book

In many ways our health depends on the health of organs located in the head and neck regions: the *brain, thyroid gland, eyes, salivary glands, ears, nose and sinuses, throat, tongue, teeth and gums.*

Besides that, our eyes, ears, mouth, and nose are the entrance gate through which air, food, water, information, thoughts, and emotions come into the body. If through these gates come unclean drink (including impure water, soft drinks, alcohol, etc.) and bad food, negative information and negative emotions, these gates, or organs, become themselves the source of infection and illness.

How to maintain these gates, and other important organs located in the head and neck region, to hold a healthy control over everything that comes through them, you will learn from this book.

This book is one in a four-part series entitled:

Healing through Cleansing.

Book 1 is about the cleansing of the main excretory organs, the colon, kidneys, lungs and skin.

Book 2 tells how to cleanse the organs located in the head and neck region, the brain, thyroid gland, eyes, salivary glands, ears, nose and sinuses, throat, tongue, teeth and gums.

Book 3 deals with cleansing the abdominal organs, the stomach, small intestine, liver, blood vessels and blood, lymph, sexual organs, joints and spine.

Book 4 presents the main principles of a healthy diet with simple recipes for preparing living food dishes and safe cooking techniques which help to prepare freshly cooked foods without losing vital nutrients. Includes a weight loss program.

Each of these books contain testimonials both in the beginning and at the end of the book.

Preface

This book is published not as a substitute for, but rather as a supplement to, the care of your professional healthcare provider. More specifically, the procedures described in this book are designed to support the body's immune system through cleansing specific internal organs and systems down to the cellular level. In this way the body can be freed from the toxins it has picked up over the years, and its natural healing capacity strengthened. The information and techniques in this book are preventative in nature for the improvement of human health.

The information and the techniques described in this book are *not* designed to provide medical consultation or advice, diagnosis, prognosis, treatment procedures or prescription of remedies for any ailment or condition as those terms might be defined or construed by any federal, state or local law, rule, regulation or ordinance. Specifically, this book is not intended to engage in anything that legally would constitute the practice of medicine. The author of this book does not claim to treat any disease or provide any cure.

Instead, the information in this book is designed to create a better understanding of how the human body is capable of taking in and storing various chemicals, waste products and unwanted biologic organisms that are detrimental to human health. Further, this book is designed to discuss the impact these have on the human body, and how their partial or complete removal is beneficial to your health. Additionally, by increasing your awareness of these processes, this book hopes to create a greater self-awareness of personal health.

Because each person is unique, the author encourages each reader to pursue a daily self-care program tailored to his or her particular situation, based on that person's own best evaluation of the circumstances and in consultation with his or her professional healthcare provider.

Contents

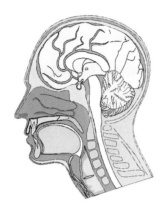

Introduction

In many ways our health depends on our lifestyle. Sometimes people who live an unhealthy lifestyle don't even know it because they don't understand what is a healthy lifestyle and what is an unhealthy lifestyle. Let's briefly describe these two ways of living.

An Unhealthy Lifestyle

An unhealthy lifestyle happens when you do not pay attention to your body and your health. People who live an unhealthy lifestyle assign either no time, or too little time, to improving their health. In addition, their diet and their lack of activity tends not toward improving health but toward

1

destroying it. An unhealthy lifestyle pollutes and weakens the whole system through the toxins it produces. Pollution to the system comes from poor diet, inactivity, poor blood and lymph circulation, lack of water and fresh air, wrong daily schedule, stresses and negative thinking, and also from the environment. Tiredness—being not just tired, but overtired, continuing to work or to work out when you feel tired, lack of rest and relaxation, and lack of sleep—is also related to an unhealthy lifestyle and increased pollution in the system.

A Healthy Lifestyle

A healthy lifestyle is the result of *the mind* having the knowledge it needs for good health, and *the will* having the wisdom and strength to implement that knowledge.

A healthy lifestyle is thinking, speaking, and acting in every way that leads to a **long life *and* high quality of living** without sacrificing any of the things in life that are truly enjoyable, profitable or natural.

A healthy lifestyle is **victory in living** not only for the physical body, but for the mind, the soul, and the spirit. As the body becomes healthier, so the mind thinks better and the soul and spirit become clearer.

A healthy lifestyle is **leaving behind the "pack mentality"** that is tragically symbolized by the lemmings that mythically race *en masse* over the proverbial cliff. It is not buying into *any* way of living that shortens your life or decreases the quality of living. It is not buying or using a product (or service) that is claimed to be good, but in reality is not. It is not allowing someone to treat your body with

2

disrespect simply because he or she needs you to buy his or her product or service.

A healthy lifestyle is a **science** wherein the healing wisdom of the ages and the advantages of state-of-the-art medical science are blended together by both the experienced health professional and the informed patient.

A healthy lifestyle is an **art form** in which, once you have achieved your health goals through natural means, you walk through life exuding good health and leading others along the same victorious path.

A healthy lifestyle includes **cleansing your body** from toxins on all levels while faithfully maintaining that cleansing by following a rational diet.

Finally, a healthy lifestyle includes learning the necessary information about **proper exercise**, developing an exercise program tailored just for you, making time for that exercise program, and then actually doing the exercises on schedule.

People who live a healthy lifestyle constantly take care not just to cleanse the external body, but also to cleanse the internal organs. All of our organs and systems down to the cellular level require regular cleansing. Nature programs our bodies for this necessary maintenance to work automatically, but for many reasons our bodies become weak and cannot do this completely by themselves. They need help.

You—the individual in control of your body—are the first and most important element in achieving the optimum health possible for your body. Once you have decided to pursue this critical goal, you will need **reliable information**.

Our Center can recommend the following books to help guide you down the path of optimum health.

1. How to help clean your organs with professional help is described in my books: *Deep Internal Body Cleansing,* and *Eight Steps to Perfect Health.*
2. How to help your own system through self-help methods is described in my books, *Healing through Cleansing, Books 1-4,* and *Unique Method of Colon Rejuvenation.*

What Are Favorable Conditions for Bacterial and Viral Reproduction?

The contemporary American diet usually includes a large number of mucus-forming foods that result in the generation of mucus throughout the body. Excess mucus often settles in the lungs, bronchi, liver, kidneys, digestive tract, and in the blood vessels. It also settles, more famously, in the head and neck organs giving rise to a number of ailments in these organs. What most people do not know is that the sinuses of the average adult can accumulate up to two (2) cups of mucus.

If an infection gets started in this mucus, the infecting bacteria or virus will start to reproduce using mucus as its food source. Mucus that has gone through the digestive process of bacteria comes out as a toxic substance.

There are certain mental and physical conditions that naturally enable bad organisms such as viruses and bacteria to grow and thrive. These include overheating, overcooling, high levels of toxic substances in the body, physical and emotional stress, depression, physical or emotional overload, etc.

If conditions favor reproduction of bacteria or viruses in the regions of head and neck, then depending on the exact location, the following problems could occur: eye infection, conjunctivitis, middle ear inflammation, sinus infection, flu, gum inflammation, headache, etc. Excess amount of mucus in sinuses, throat, bronchi and lungs can be activated by smells, plant pollen, and foods to which one is allergic. These provoke an allergic reactions such as tearing, eye redness, allergic cold, inflamed throat or nose, allergic cough, asthmatic cough, etc.

To get rid of high levels of toxicity in the whole body, including excess mucus in the head and neck organs, you must undergo a series of cleansings of the large and small intestine plus the liver, and adjust your diet. But to regularly maintain your body in good shape you have to take care of it every day. Right down to the teeth.

To learn more about unique cleansing procedures done in our center, please visit our website at
www.koyfmancenter.com

"Difficulties with Breathing, Depression, Bad Sleeping, and Muscle Pain"

I had difficulties with breathing, depression, bad sleeping, and muscle pain. When I started my treatment in Dr. Koyfman's office, my health became much better even from the first visit. My sleeping became better. I have a good mood and good spirit! I stopped taking any medications. Of course it is a long way for me to drive from South Carolina, but it is worth it! I will continue my treatment to be completely healthy.
Thank you very much, Dr. Koyfman, for everything you are doing for your patients.
 May God bless you.   Darya Djebelli

Brain Fog

Ever since I had my baby, 5 years ago, I have not been "normal". Constant lack of energy, forgetfulness and bad mood. I haven't been able to be good a mother or wife. I came across one of Dr. Koyfman's books and it changed my life. I started applying his techniques to my daily routine and felt a huge difference. Then I decided to try his actual cleansing procedures and Oh, My God! I am reborn. My memory is great. I think clearly. My energy level jumped through the roof. I finally lost all the "baby weight". It turned out that everything was caused by the candida overgrowth and hormonal dissbalance. Dr. Koyfman was very knowledgeable in this matter and helped me very quickly. I am finally able to enjoy my family and not scared to have more kids.
My whole life style changed and I am glad that now I can teach it to my kids.   --Rita K. N.Y, N.Y

6

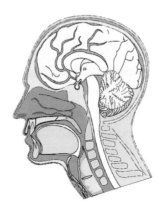

Brain

How Negative Thoughts and Emotions Affect the Brain

In the course of each human life innumerable stresses in the form of fears and negative emotions pass through him or her, leaving their marks in the form of tension in internal organs, muscles, glands and blood vessels. Some of these stresses begin before birth.

But before these emotions write themselves onto these different parts of the body, they leave their imprints on that part of the brain that corresponds to that individual organ, muscle, gland or system. As a result, the brain is affected by

7

each of these emotional stresses regardless of whether they are small or large.

This emotional refuse—left behind in the brain and the rest of the body—is a form of pollution that can have a significant effect on a person's health. The tensions left behind can form barriers throughout the body and the brain. **These barriers isolate the brain from different parts of the body so that the brain loses the precise control that it had over the various organs, etc.** When we lose any of the control between the brain and other organs, the result is destroyed function of body organs and therefore an increase in various diseases.

This emotional refuse and its effects on the body are compounded and renewed by every new stress that comes into our individual lives. And this world is full of incredible stresses and tensions from the everyday problems of work, traffic, unhappy people, etc., to larger issues such as the economy and conflicts in other nations that overflow in the form of air planes and skyscrapers.

Old and new tensions consume an enormous amount of our physical, emotional and spiritual energy. They also block the flow of physical, emotional and spiritual energy in the brain and the body. This interferes with the vital transport of blood, nutrients, lymph fluids, tissue fluids, and oxygen. It also interferes with the natural flow of energy throughout the human system.

Tensions can exist in the body either in a dormant or in an active state. When the tensions are dormant, we seem to cope fairly well with these tensions and the blockages that they cause. Their harmful influence on the body is inflicted slowly (chronic). But when the tensions are active the body starts to feel significant overloads that can lead to a serious disorder or illness.

Recurrence of tensions can be provoked by new stresses; poisoning by food, air water or medicines; overheating; alcohol; overwork and other factors. **The lessening or even elimination of tensions and their consequences (the pollution of the body with emotional refuse) is an important key to health and happiness physically, emotionally and spiritually.**

It is impossible to separate cleansing the body of emotional refuse from cleansing the brain of the same. *The human organism is a cumulative, holistic system, and everything in it is connected to the brain. Thus, the cleansing of the organs of emotional refuse affects the brain, and the cleansing of the brain of emotional refuse affects the rest of the body.* The same is true of cleansing of physical toxins.

Methods of Brain Cleansing

Any discussion of brain cleansing inevitably leads to jokes concerning "brainwashing." Fortunately, this is as far as that connection goes. Jokes. The techniques of brain cleansing discussed here do not include any form of brainwashing by any definition. These methods do not include altering the mind or its perceptions with chemicals, political ideology or anything from the Cold War or Madison Avenue. The closest you will get to brainwashing is when you close this book and turn on the television. There you will find a host of "brainwashing" commercials designed to make you believe that their unnatural food product is somehow "OK."

Methods of cleansing the brain involve improving blood circulation and activating the brain centers responsible for the various organs through massage, exercises, diet, conscious relaxation, meditation and removal of toxins. **All of these methods will improve connection between the brain and all other organs and increase control from the brain over the whole organism**. Some of these techniques are described below.

Cleansing the Organs and Systems

Cleansing the various organs and systems of the human body of the different toxins that have been stored in it. This includes cleansing the large intestine, the liver, the kidneys, the lymph system, blood vessels, the blood and the brain.

Cleansing the Nose and Sinuses

The cleansing of nasal sinuses improves the quality of respiration, increases the amount of oxygen that gets into the brain, which makes the brain healthier and improves the clarity of thought.

Yoga Respiratory Exercises

The respiratory exercises of yoga also facilitate a greater flow of oxygen into the brain.

Therapeutic Walking

Therapeutic walking is one of the simplest and most effective methods for improving the health of the whole body and the brain in particular. Methods 2, 3 and 4 facilitate the enrichment of the brain with oxygen. Oxygen is a very important nutrient for the brain. It also facilitates the neutralization of toxins and their evacuation from the body. But excess oxygen can be toxic. The symptoms that point to an excessive intake of oxygen include dizziness and weakness. That is why you should be moderate with respiratory exercises.

Improving Circulation in the Neck

All blood vessels that supply the brain with nutrients pass through the neck. Improving the circulation in the vicinity of the neck leads to better circulation in the brain. You can improve circulation in the neck with exercises and massage for it. For descriptions of massage techniques and neck exercises, see the chapter about the throat in this book. Further descriptions of neck exercises are given in my book, *Unique Method of Colon Rejuvenation.*

Scalp Massage

Massage of the scalp also improves the circulation in the brain.

Massage and Exercises for the Temples, Ears, and Eyes

Massage of the temples, the ears and the eyes and exercises for the eyes reflexively improve the circulation of blood in the brain. This improves the brain's connection and control over the rest of the body.

Yoga Upside-down Poses

The upside-down poses of yoga facilitate a greater flow of blood towards the brain. This activates circulation in the brain and facilitates the cleansing of its blood vessels.

Using a Slant Board

The use of a slant board eases the completion of the upside-down poses of yoga. Also, you can simply lie on the slant board, completely relaxed, and still get its positive effects.

Therapeutic Effects of Exercises on a Slant Board

- Increases brain circulation.
- Improves the connection between the brain and organs.
- Improves the circulation and function of the thyroid gland.
- Helps release gas blockages in the small and large intestines.
- Helps overcome constipation.
- Activate abdominal breathing, which helps improve circulation in the liver, pancreas, stomach, small intestine and other organs.
- Helps return digestive organs to their normal position after having sagged down onto the reproductive organs from being overloaded with food and waste.
- Decrease pain in leg veins, which helps prevent varicose veins and cellulite.
- Helps cure hemorrhoids.
- Improves circulation in the face, improves the color of the skin and softens wrinkles.
- Improves vision and hearing.
- Relaxes and rests the heart.
- Improves your thinking.

12

Fasting

Fasting powerfully cleanses and strengthens the vessels of the brain. To see how you can correctly conduct a fast, see my book, *Eight Steps to Perfect Health.*

Exercises and Massages

Exercises and massages facilitate the softening and liquidation of tensions in the body, the organs and the brain.

Mental Focus

Deliberately focusing the power of the mind on areas of tension, and consciously relaxing them, will significantly decrease or even eliminate their tension.

Meditation

There are many methods of meditation. They are described in books on yoga, tai-chi, Zen, etc. The simplest kind of meditation is when you sit relaxed, with a straight back, and direct your gaze into yourself. This means that you listen to things that happen inside your body. When your attention passes over tensions, which, hold imprints of your negative emotions, fears, grudges, traumas etc., it might happen that your attention will prompt "playback" of the negative emotion recorded on the tense region. And you will start to feel and suffer it again. If you allow this to happen without interfering with this process, without suppressing it, the negative emotion in this area or organ will go away and the tension will disappear. Sometimes you might feel fear, reluctance to go through the unpleasant event again; do not submit to this fear. Relive the event, but don't take it to heart. There is nothing you can do now. After all, it was in the past. You only need to look at it from a different angle. That is a reliable way to get rid of harmful emotions and tensions.

Positive Thinking

There are people who are optimistic by nature. They almost always think positively and hope for the best. *Positive thinking protects the brain and other organs against the harmful effects of negative thoughts, emotions or tensions.* Regardless of how optimistic you are naturally, you can always improve this disposition. **The first step** is to want to have a lifestyle of positive thinking. **The second step** is to decide to *begin and continue* thinking positively. (This is done by deciding to assume the best whenever reasonable, and to strongly consider the most positive aspect of any situation.) **The third step** is to implement this thinking as often as you can. Do not berate yourself if you fail. Instead, consider the most positive aspect of the situation by remembering that you want the best for yourself and that you are pursuing it. Keep working on it until it becomes natural.

Controlling the Thoughts

The way our life goes is the result of our thoughts— unfortunately, often chaotic and negative. Organising, controlling and programming your thoughts can improve the quality of your life.

Resting the Brain

Our brain is constantly loaded with thoughts. There are so many of them that they don't give any rest to either the brain or the body. *It is not hard to prove that thinking uses energy.* Everyone can remember an event when you pondered some difficult problem while sitting passively in a chair, and then felt exhausted, often even more so than after physical work. Like all parts of the body, the brain needs rest. Wholesome sleep provides the brain with good rest. Another way to let the brain rest is to free it of thought for a while. How to do that is described in the chapter about the role of the mind in Book 1 of this series, *Healing through Cleansing.*

Feeding the Energy of the Immune System

The Energy Principle of Fighting Disease. Having established that thought consumes energy, we should also realize that thought also transforms energy from one form of energy to another. The same principle is found in the science of physics as stated in the Law of Conservation of Energy and Matter. Therefore, we should not be surprised if this same principle is found elsewhere in the natural world.

The human organism consumes the energy of the universe from the Sun, the Moon, and the stars, plus the energy of food, water and air, which also get their energy from the Sun, the Moon and the stars. We eat this food and our system transforms this energy into different kinds of energy, such as chemical, electrical, magnetic, mechanical, and thermal. *The process of thought is the result of all of these types of energy, i.e., thought is the overall energy of the organism.*

Thought can also produce various types of energy depending on the type of thinking that is occurring. For example if you are pondering a negative emotion (envy, jealousy, bitterness, hate, unrighteous anger, etc.) that kind of energy is produced. If on the other hand you are contemplating a *positive emotion (love, happiness, joy, etc.) you generate that kind of energy.* **If**

15

you think negatively, you create destructive energy. If you think positively, you create constructive energy. Often the choice is yours because thoughts can be controlled.

To understand how one can use thought to heal, let us look at the following example:

As a result of a poor diet, toxins, stresses and other harmful factors a man got sick. He feels pain and weakness. There are two kinds of energy in such a man. One kind is the energy of the disease (toxins, parasites, tensions). The other kind of energy is the energy of the immune system, which tries to neutralise and eliminate the toxins from the organism. In other words *there is a constant, deadly war between the two kinds of energy in the body: the energy of the disease and the energy of the body's defences.*

So how is the outcome of this war affected by the third kind of energy, the energy of thought? If, by submitting to the energy of the disease, we begin to think about bad things, i.e. what unpleasant outcome the disease may have, we produce energy that aids the disease. How does that happen?

On one hand, such thinking creates the emotion of fear. Fear constrains and constricts all vital pathways of an organism - blood and lymph vessels, digestive organs, endocrine glands, etc. Furthermore, nutrition and cleansing of organs and systems are disturbed even more. And that, of course, reinforces the disease's energy.

On the other hand, such thinking programs the body, i.e. records on the brain, muscles and other organs a *program of destruction.* If this type of thinking is constantly present, eventually this program will run.

But since we can control our thoughts, we can start to think positively, and program health into our minds and our bodies.

16

It doesn't matter that you're weak right now. **Positive thinking will feed the energy of the immune system.**

There are many techniques for reinforcing the energy of our defence system using thought. Let us name one such method.

Programmed Suggestion

The idea behind this method is in programming your mind for positive emotions. For example, suppose you caught a cold and feel pain in your throat and head, you feel weak, perhaps you have a fever, etc. This condition leads to a lot of toxic mucus and pathogens collecting in your body and your immune system waging war with the disease. If you use "programmed suggestion" in this situation, it will produce energy that helps your immune system in its war with the disease.

Here are the approximate formulas for such suggestion:

"My brain is perfectly interconnected with every organ, gland, system and fiber in my body. My head is light and clear. My throat is perfectly healthy. I am perfectly healthy. My body has ultimate immunity against any disease or illness." Repeat this for 5 to 10 minutes, several times daily. **Positive formulas** such as the above **produce positive thinking which produces positive energy.** The words *"perfect and absolute"* create an emotional background that strengthens this energy even more. You can strengthen it still further by *clearly visualising* what you are thinking or talking about.

The greatest amount of healing energy will be produced when you not only say these words, but also **absolutely believe** that they will work. And belief comes when you have knowledge and understanding of this process.

"Positive Suggestion" is one of the most wonderful methods of healing the brain.

Starving the Energy of the Disease

Of course, you should help your body fight disease not only with "Positive Suggestion," but also with all other known natural methods. **You can weaken the energy of disease by doing the following:**

1. Cleansing the colon and removing the negative energy of toxins from it;
2. Cleansing the stomach to remove the negative energy of toxins from it;
3. Cleansing the skin by means of a shower and opening its pores to help remove poisons through the skin, or perhaps taking a sauna or drinking diuretic tea to help the kidneys;
4. Not loading the body with foods that require a lot of energy for digestion.

This list could be continued, but it is beyond the scope of this section.

Protecting the Head

One more simple truth: The head, and thus the brain, must be protected against heat, cold and physical shocks.

Sustaining your brain in a cleansed, healthy state is a vital key to good health, clear thought, success in life and happiness.

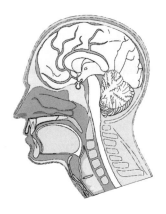

Teeth and Gums

Functions of the Teeth

The first organs of the digestive tract are the teeth. They are used to break down food physically to increase its surface area. The greater the surface area of the food, the more accessible food is to the chemical actions of saliva and stomach juices. This chemical action is vital to digesting food to get the maximum amount of nutrients from the food and to generate the least amount of waste from its digestion.

The problem is that today we are always in a hurry, and often do not take the time to carefully chew our food. Many of us swallow our food in chunks not thinking about the role of teeth and saliva in digestion. People act as if the goal is to throw down their food, and then the rest will follow automatically.

During chewing two things happen. **First,** the food in your mouth becomes saturated with saliva to make it ready (chemically) for digestion in the stomach. **Second,** the teeth break down the molecular structure of the food to release biological energy contained in intermolecular bonds and in the molecules themselves. The more the food gets broken down the more energy is released. This released energy starts to become consumed in the mouth through tongue and epiglottal nerves, and continues to be consumed in the stomach and in the small intestine. **Those who chew their food better receive more energy and nutrition, and consequently eat less.**

Therefore, if you don't chew your food properly you are (1) losing a large part of its energy content, (2) do not experience the maximum satisfaction from chewing, (3) tend to overeat, and (4) will make your stomach do extra work needlessly.

Because the stomach does not have teeth and cannot physically break down food, it has to compensate for the deficiency of poor chewing by increasing the acidity of stomach juices. (If you have ever had acid indigestion or any other problem caused by excessive acidity in the stomach, you know what pain this can cause.) Increased acidity will either lead to damage of the stomach wall (ulcers), or to depleting stomach acids so that the stomach can not maintain the necessary acidity for digestion. If this happens, foods will not properly digest, leading to decreased nutrients being absorbed and unnecessary waste being created.

That's why proper chewing is a very important chemical (saturation with saliva) and physical (release of molecular energy) process for the body. **Chewing is the only consciously controlled process in digestion,** so it is up to you to do it correctly. But to properly chew and break down food it is necessary to have healthy teeth.

Structure of the Teeth

Teeth are hard, bony structures located in the jaw. Each tooth consists of two main parts: coronas covered with enamel, and roots growing inside the jaw. Inside of each tooth there is an empty space containing pulp. Pulp is a very sensitive, light tissue which contains blood and lymph vessels, plus nerves coming to the tooth through little openings at the base of the root. Pulp is covered by a dense substance, dentin, making up the largest part of the tooth.

Gums are made up of dense, meaty tissue covering the part of the jaw, which contains teeth.

If we don't take good care of teeth and gums they could become infected with different bacteria, resulting in decay processes, which will poison and weaken the whole body. Lets briefly look at what kind of problems can result if we do not take care of them and will not follow a healthy diet.

Bleeding Gums

This particular malady can be caused by a variety of things, such as too much pressure from a toothbrush. There are also infectious diseases of the gums. Gingivitis is a gum infection where gums become inflamed, red, mushy, and bleed easily. In other, more serious gum infections, puss can forms in the space between teeth and gums.

Toothache

The pain most people feel in their teeth is the result of tooth decay, and can be exacerbated by foods that are too sweet or too cold. If tooth pain is caused by heat, then the pulp has been injured and an abscess can form. Tooth decay can also occur when the teeth are not properly cleansed and some food remains on the surface of the teeth. This food, especially sweet and sticky foods, stick to the surface of the teeth and get stuck between them. These food particles start to decay, with the help of parasite infection, and release acid, which chemically attacks the enamel and gradually damages it enough to get to the dentin, which also starts to degrade.

Mercury Fillings

For approximately 175 years, dentists have been filling cavities in people's teeth with an amalgamation of silver, mercury and other metals. These fillings are often 50% mercury, 25% silver, and the rest often composed of tin, copper, zinc and other materials. Because the color of this material is roughly silver in color, dentists call them "silver fillings." However, the dental professionals will never mention that these fillings contain mercury. In fact, the American Dental Association warns dental professionals to use extreme caution when handling dental amalgam for the short time they handle it. Yet the estimated 85% of Americans that have these fillings have them in their mouths (unprotected) 24 hours per day for the rest of their lives.

When you stop to think for a minute about the physical and chemical characteristics of mercury, you have to wonder why the dental profession ever felt comfortable putting something as dangerous as mercury in our teeth. Mercury is liquid at room temperature. In fact it is liquid at most any temperature that humans can survive in. Additionally, a puddle of mercury just sitting out in the open will volatilize at room or mouth temperature. This means it will release molecules of mercury into the surrounding air without any provocation. If you heat it, even more mercury molecules are released into the surrounding environment.

The temperature of foods and beverages that we sometimes put into our mouths can be more than twice our normal body temperature. This rise in temperature in the mouth and teeth tends to cause the mercury fillings to release more mercury than they normally would. Once released, the mercury mixes with whatever food or beverage we have in our mouths and is swallowed. It has now left its storage in the fillings and has entered our personal body chemistry.

Mercury, if you did not happen to know it, is a very poisonous chemical. The World Health Organization and other leading health entities have stated that there is no known level of mercury that is safe in the human body. No government agency has ever put it on any list of nutrients, or said there is a "recommended daily allowance" for mercury. Quite the opposite. The Environmental Protection Agency has officially declared that mercury is a hazardous waste when discarded.

Just some of the many bad things mercury can do to the body are: (1) kills off the good bacteria in the small and large intestines creating a hospitable environment for parasites, (2) weakens the immune system, and (3) interferes with protein absorption. The list goes on and on. Entire books have been devoted to issue of mercury fillings. To make matters even worse, the metals the dentists have put in our teeth can not only conduct electricity, but can form a "battery" effect in our mouths between the saliva and the mercury. This unnatural electrical environment in the mouth can disrupt the natural energy flow through the body's meridians.

To get rid of these fillings requires a dental professional who appreciates the problem, and is experienced in removing mercury amalgam dental fillings. Improper removal can be more dangerous than leaving the fillings there. **Whether you choose to have these heavy metal fillings removed or not, it is still a wise idea to cleanse the mercury and other unwanted metals from your body through deep internal body cleansing.** This includes colon cleansing, and (especially important) small intestine cleansing and liver cleansing. We do all of these procedures in our center and achieve good results with removal of heavy metals.

Meanwhile, you will still want to prevent damage to your teeth and infections by performing certain daily actions for their good health.

Yoga Methods of Teeth Care

Yoga does not advocate the use toothbrushes or toothpaste. Instead, Yoga practitioners use little twigs from the Neem tree. (Twigs from the eucalyptus and oak tree are acceptable as well.) Twigs to be used for cleaning teeth should be cut in the Spring, and they should be 6 to 8 inches (15 to 20 cm) long with a diameter of approximately an eighth to a quarter inch (3-5 mm). After being cut, the twigs are dried.

The Twig Method

For daily use, a twig is put in a cup of clean, cold water in the evening. The next morning, the end of the soaked twig is softened with the teeth until a little brush is formed on that end. This brush is then used to brush the teeth and to massage the gums. After you finish brushing your teeth with the twig, cut off the brush end of the twig and save the twig for the next "tooth brushing." This way one twig will last several times. The twig method is performed every other day. The following procedure is used between teeth brushing with twigs.

The Salt Method

Take fine sea salt and add olive oil. Mix these two until a viscous paste is formed. After thoroughly washing your hands, put some of this paste on your thumb and index finger to massage your teeth and gums for 2 to 3 minutes. Make sure you massage both sides of your gums, and avoid excessive pressure on your gums, especially in the beginning when you are not used to it. **Salt is a wonderful disinfectant in that it kills bacteria and fungus and thereby strengthens the teeth and gums. With the help of this simple paste you can "treat" such serious conditions as peridontitis and others similar afflictions.** This procedure is also great for cleaning teeth enamel because salt works like sand paper. Just be careful and don't overdo it.

But brushing only in the morning is not sufficient to maintain the health of your gums and teeth. Since we eat and drink a wide variety of foods and beverages during the day there is time for food particles to get stuck on and between our teeth, and on our gums. Even if you eat the healthiest diet, this is still a problem. This is because decay and fermentation of this food is a very fast process, especially if some bacteria got into your mouth along with the food.

To prevent damage to teeth, and to prevent gum infection, it is important to rinse out your mouth after every meal and after every drink (unless you are drinking water). Water temperature should be warm. During that time it would also be beneficial to lightly massage your teeth and gums with your thumb and index fingers for 10 to 20 seconds. (Wash your hands properly first!) This massage will help remove essentially all of the food particles on your teeth and gums, and will improve blood circulation in gums and teeth.

The quality of the food you eat also affects the health of gums and teeth. A large role in maintaining healthy teeth is played by raw vegetables, which deliver a lot of necessary vitamins and minerals, and also provide good exercise for your teeth. This is because the process of chewing is in itself a good stimulator of blood circulation in teeth and gums.

Daosk Method

This is a simple, painless method of strengthening the teeth and activating circulation in the teeth and gums. It does not require any special equipment to perform this procedure. You should not do this procedure, or its variant, if you feel any significant pain, or if your dental professional recommends that you do not do these procedures.

First, put your top and bottom teeth together. Press them together lightly in a position where they naturally fit together. Now, separate your top set of teeth from your lower set of teeth by lowering your bottom jaw. Keep your lips sealed. By moving your bottom jaw, start lightly tapping your bottom teeth against your upper teeth. You will hear a slight sound as you do this. Perform this light tapping of the teeth about 10 to 15 times. You should consider doing this procedure twice a day. Gradually increase the number of taps to 20 to 30 or more times. The therapeutic effects of this simple procedure come from increasing the flow of blood in the gums and teeth.

Daosk Variant

Put your bottom and top teeth together carefully using moderate pressure. Hold the pressure for three to four seconds then relax. Repeat 5 to 10 or more times. This exercise is also excellent for improving blood flow and preventing stagnant conditions favorable to bacterial infection growth.

Koyfman Method

Use natural toothpaste in a plastic tube. Squeeze all the toothpaste out into a disposable cup. Add 30-50% fine-grained seal salt. Mix carefully with a disposable spoon.

Use a special large syringe available at the Koyfman Center. Remove the plunger and fill the barrel through the plunger opening with the toothpaste-salt mixture. Cover the plunger rubber with olive oil. Insert the plunger into the barrel and depress it to expel all air.

Squeeze all air out of the empty toothpaste tube. Put the tip of the syringe to the mouth of the toothpaste tube and depress the syringe plunger to insert the new toothpaste-salt mixture into the toothpaste tube. Clean syringe for the next use.

The toothpaste is now ready for use as usual. At the beginning, brush gently until the gums strengthen; then brush more firmly.

Natural toothpaste mixed with sea salt has increased disinfectant and cleansing properties. With this paste you may clean your teeth with a brush or with your finger. I usually do both, first brushing the teeth and gums, then massaging the gums with my fingers. Be sure to rinse the mouth with clean water after using toothpaste.

Food Good for Your Teeth

Some foods are just better for your dental health than others. These foods include: fresh fruits and vegetables, onion, garlic, radish, fresh fruit and vegetable juices, oatmeal, nuts, seeds, fresh greens, and some herbs that grow in the wild.

Food Harmful for Your Teeth

Just as some foods are the "good guys," other foods are the villains. The foods that are bad for your dental health include sugar and all sugar products such as candy, cakes, pies, cookies, jellies, jams, and all beverages containing sugar. Sharp changes in temperature of consumed foods or beverages are also harmful because this thermal shock damages tooth enamel.

Modern Methods of Teeth Care

I am not advocating that anyone stop cleansing their teeth in the traditional manner with a toothbrush and with toothpaste. If you choose to utilize this method, just remember that there are certain things you need to do to get the most out of this technique and to prevent some of the problems that are inherent with the traditional toothbrush.

First, wash your toothbrush carefully after each use. If you fail to do this, food particles will remain trapped in the bristles of your brush. Certainly you can see some such food particles, but the vast majority are too small to be visible to the naked eye. These trapped food particles provide food for bacteria to grow, and such an uncleansed toothbrush can re-introduce those old food particles (and bacteria) back into your mouth. Bacteria can be a source of infection. Also, **never store your toothbrush in a case.** The conditions there are very favorable for the growth of bacteria.

Natural toothpastes are available in health stores, which are safe to use. You can combine modern methods with those described above and achieve satisfactory results.

Garlic

That "wonder herb" known as garlic has a very beneficial application for your mouth's health. The procedure is simple and powerful. In the evening, after you have finished eating for the day and have already brushed your teeth, take one fresh raw clove of garlic and peel it with your already carefully washed hands. Put the garlic in your mouth and chew it slowly, moving the chewed pulp all around your mouth. Then spit it out. In a few minutes rinse out your mouth with clean water. Be advised that this is a powerful technique since garlic contains some powerful chemicals. Because of the strong taste of garlic, some people will not be able to chew garlic.

About this time the average reader is saying, "Whoa! That is gonna burn my mouth, and it will run people away from me." Granted, when you first chew raw, fresh garlic it might create a burning sensation in your mouth, but if you do the procedure regularly the sensation will go away. Yes, you will get used to it. As for the anti-social smell of garlic, don't let the smell stop you. The smell you get from decaying food and infection in the mouth is much worse than the natural smell of garlic. If you are concerned with the smell try chewing 2 to 3 parsley stems to make the smell. **Remember,** garlic is an excellent natural antibiotic; no infection can withstand direct contact with garlic.

29

Just ask yourself which you would rather have in your mouth: the taste of garlic or the taste of an infection. It your choice.

First Aid for Tooth Pain

If you have strong or serious tooth pain, it means that you have infection in your teeth or gums and you need to see a dentist.

While waiting to see your dentist, you can easily kill the infection and relieve the pain by doing the following:

- Use 1 c. (8 oz.) warm, clean water.
- Add 2 tsp. sea salt and stir until dissolved.
- Sip a little of the solution and swish it forcefully around the affected area.
- Hold the solution in your mouth as long as you can and then spit it out.
- Continue until the cup is empty.

This will kill infection and relieve pain. Repeat the steps every 1-2 hours until the pain is completely stopped.

When the pain stops, you may think you don't want to go to the dentist, but do not neglect this. You still need to see your dentist.

Conclusion: If we want to have healthy teeth, it is not enough to go to the dentist. It is necessary to take care of your teeth everyday and even several times a day.

When we have decayed teeth and inflamed gums, it means that we have infections (parasites) in our mouth which not only destroy teeth and gums but, together with food and saliva, goes into the digestive system and the blood. There these infections continue to develop in more serious stages to destroy digestion and poison the blood.

Infection in the teeth and gums could be the beginning of many health problems, including serious situations like sinus problems, heart disorders, digestive problems, blood and lymph disorders, and even cancer.

Keeping the teeth and gums clean and healthy protects us from disease not only in these organs but also in the whole body.

"I Suddenly Stopped Having Difficulty in Breathing"

I met Yakov Koyfman on the day he came to Atlanta. I helped him and his family as they took their first steps in America. That was the extent of my involvement with them at that time.

Approximately one year later I was diagnosed with asthma. The traditional doctors I was seeing at the time said they couldn't promise to cure me since asthma is not a curable disease. Then I remembered Dr. Koyfman after seeing his advertisement in a newspaper. I called him up on the telephone, and refreshed his memory about me. When I told Dr. Koyfman about my asthma he said that he would try his best to help me. He said that I would have to patiently follow his directions and agree to go through his fasting program. I resisted, saying that fasting was prohibited for me because I had discovered fasting caused me headaches, and if started

31

eating again my pain will go away. I ended up not choosing to follow his program.

Another year went by and I went to the hospital with an asthma attack. Then my daughter actually forced me to go to Dr. Koyfman for help. I began fasting according to his instructions. For 21 days I had only water and fresh juice. I tried to walk a lot, but I had difficulty breathing. At the end of this fast I took another 21 days to slowly and carefully come off of the fast by eating minimally according to Dr. Koyfman's instructions. I could see and feel that I had lost weight, but strangely felt more energetic and stronger. I suddenly stopped having difficulty in breathing during walking, even for long distances.

Although I had never complained about my liver, Dr. Koyfman suggested a "liver cleanse." I agreed because by now I had come to trust his advice. How surprised I was when I saw how many stones my "healthy" liver discarded.

Now another year has gone by and I feel normal. I no longer have to limit my food and best of all I don't have headaches or difficulty breathing. I feel active, strong, and young. For me it is simply a miracle. I cannot find another word for it. And Dr. Koyfman is the author of this miracle. I am very appreciative of his skills, experience and knowledge. He became for me a most special person. I thank him very much.

- Irina (Esfir) Gilmer, Daytona Beach, Florida

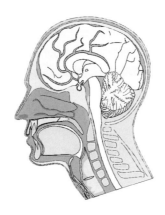

Tongue

The tongue is a most unique organ. In humans it is so powerful that it is the beginning and ending of most wars, and the death of many peoples' reputations and feelings. The tongue, with its unquenchable appetite for pleasure in the form of "what tastes good," is an organ that gets many people into trouble not just in terms of speech, but in its voracious desire for the wrong foods. Too often this small, wayward organ influences or moves the whole body in much the same manner as that old saying about the tail wagging the dog.

That bit of moralizing aside, the tongue, in any animal, is a muscle that is housed in a moist cavity of the head, covered with a thin mucus membrane, and is occasionally exposed to the outside elements. It is important to notice that this singular organ is not smooth on its upper exterior. Because of its somewhat rough topside, it has the unfortunate habit of collecting food particles, bits of mucus, and way too many types and numbers of bacteria and viruses. Like the rest of the body, it needs to be kept clean, or diseases and other sicknesses may result.

These characteristics are just one more reason why we need to chew our food properly. When we chew our food we release moisture stored in the food, and simultaneously stimulate the release of saliva. Moisture from these two sources naturally moisten the tongue and improve the taste of food. (The tongue can not taste when it is dry.) This moisture is also important in helping us swallow our food easily so that we are not as likely to choke.

The tongue, along with saliva, is the very beginning of the digestive process. While the tongue helps to move food around in our mouths for better chewing (physical breakdown), saliva begins breaking down our food into its necessary components for further digestion (chemical breakdown). Everything that happens in the digestive system is affected by the tongue and saliva.

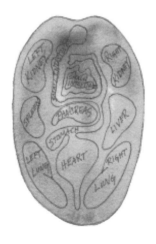

"Popping the Hood"

To better understand this diminutive organ you can begin by simply opening your mouth and taking a look at it in the mirror.

Color

If your tongue is a pale color, you may have the symptoms of anemia, or a reduced amount of blood in your body.

If your tongue is yellowish, then you may have excess bile in your gall bladder, or an imbalance in the functioning of the liver.

If your tongue is bluish (assuming you haven't eaten anything that would make it blue), it may mean that you have heart problems.

Morphological Characteristics

If you have a thin membrane covering your tongue it may mean that there are significant toxins in your digestive system.

If the membrane covers only the back part of your tongue it may mean that the toxins are predominantly in the large intestine.

If you see teeth prints on the edges of your tongue that suggests a problem with absorbing food in the intestines.

A line in the middle of your tongue may mean spinal problems. If this line is curved it might mean that the spine is misaligned.

Timing

It is better to explore your tongue in the morning before consuming any food or drink because later in the day we "eat" the membrane from our tongue. Because of this we can get a more accurate picture of the tongue's health in the morning. You can get even more information from your tongue during fasting. This is because the walls of digestive tract become exposed and can more accurately reflect internal conditions in the tongue.

How You Can Cleanse Your Organs from Toxicity and Improve Their Function with Tongue Cleansing

Instead of eating the toxins that invariably accumulate on the tongue and sending them down into our bodies, we need to remove them to decrease the overall level of toxicity in the body. There are many different methods of tongue cleansing. Here are just a few of them.

Spoon Method

Take a teaspoon, preferably made of silver. First determine if the spoon is correct for this procedure by touching its edges with your finger. If the edges are too sharp you may end up hurting your tongue. If the edges are too dull you won't be able to properly clean your tongue. A little common sense and a dash of intuition will be very helpful here. Now, rinse out your mouth with good, clean water. Take your spoon and use the edges to scrape your tongue with little, light movements starting from the root and going towards the tip. After a few motions you will see a membrane of toxicity on the spoon. Wash the spoon with water. Continue scraping your tongue and washing the spoon until you are sure that the tongue is clean. Rinse out your mouth with clean water.

36

Toothbrush Method

Instead of a spoon you can use a toothbrush with soft, natural fibers. Remember that the bristles of a toothbrush can retain or harbor some of the toxins and bacteria you brush from your tongue. Since the bristles of a toothbrush are more difficult to cleanse than the edge of a spoon, you should exercise great care and diligence in cleaning the bristles after each use. You should also be careful how you store your toothbrush so that bacteria do not grow on the bristles while the toothbrush is not in use. For example, never store your toothbrush in a case. The conditions there (moist and dark) are very favorable for the growth of bacteria.

Auverdic Method

In health stores you can find special auverdic scrapers for tongue cleansing. They are easier to use than the two preceding methods, and if you find one I recommend that you use it. They work the same way as a teaspoon. Start from the root of the tongue and move towards the tip. The mouth should be open wide, and the tongue should be sticking out. If you practice in front of the mirror you will master this procedure a lot faster.

Warning. Do not overdo it. Do not scrape your tongue too much or you may cause irritation. In case you do end up with irritation, put some (cool) melted butter or olive oil on your tongue and let it sit there without swallowing.

Finger Massage Method

Open your mouth and stick out your tongue. Using your index finger and the middle finger of one hand, lightly massage the top of your tongue with these two fingers using both circular and up and down motions. This will stimulate the circulation in this organ helping it to circulate out toxins inside of your tongue. (Try not to trigger your gag reflex. If you start coughing or feel nauseated, stop the procedure, spit out any saliva, rinse out your mouth, and continue massaging your tongue. Because you should be practicing this procedure in the morning prior to eating, there is less of a chance of feeling nauseated since your stomach is empty.)

Caution. Before you attempt this method, please understand that the hands, particularly the fingers, are a major way in which we come in contact with our world. Because of this, the fingers can be one of the dirtiest parts of the human body. Under the fingernails is often the filthiest and the hardest to clean. Please exercise the greatest and most diligent care in cleaning the fingers and under the nails before putting your fingers in your mouth. Also, your fingernails should be cut short for this technique.

Therapeutic Cough

When you clean your tongue with your finger, after several massage movements, lightly press with your fingers on your tongue. This pressure will create a light cough.

As with sneezing, nature uses coughing to cleanse the lungs, bronchi, and throat from excessive mucus, dust, pollen and bacteria. A cough usually begins with an irritation in the throat. Then we automatically inhale a deep breath and for a moment we hold the breath. This holding of the breath creates muscle tightness in the abdominal area, in the chest and throat, and also in the internal organs located in these areas: lungs, bronchi, stomach, liver, thyroid, etc.

After holding the breath we produce a fast and strong exhalation together with the coughing, and during this exhalation our system eliminates mucus, bacteria, pollen, etc.

The fast muscle contraction and relaxation in the upper body improves blood and lymph circulation in all organs in the abdominal area and in the chest, head, and neck.

But we don't need to wait until we get ill and nature initiates coughing to eliminate toxins, because toxins, dust, and pollen come into the system every day. It is better to create the coughing artificially 2-3 times every day while you clean your tongue. This simple procedure doesn't take time and it will prevent a lot of problems.

After each coughing you need to clean your throat with clean water, or even better with salt water. This simple procedure has many benefits which reach far beyond the cleansing of the pulmonary system.

Therapeutic Effects of Tongue Cleansing and Therapeutic Coughing

These simple tongue cleansing procedures can yield a variety of benefits:

• Cleanses the tongue of toxic substances.
• Activates the work of internal organs which correspond to different regions of the tongue. This is because different parts of the tongue are connected to different parts of the body through meridians (energetic channels).

- Removes mucus from your throat.
- Activates blood flow through thyroid and parathyroid glands.
- Spasmatic vibrations of the stomach from therapeutic coughing help in its cleansing and improve digestion.
- Improves functioning of the liver and the pancreas because stomach vibrations get passed on to those organs.
- When you cough you will also notice that your eyes become moist. This happens because toxic substances are removed from the eyes via tears, which means that the procedure also cleanses the eyes and can help prevent eye infection.
- Increases blood circulation in the neck and head area, cleansing and improving blood vessels in the brain, which makes them more flexible.
- If in the morning on waking, you feel sleepy, this simple procedure will wake you up completely, and you will feel refreshed and clear headed.

Tongue Exercises

No doubt many who read these words will be thinking to themselves that the average person does not need to exercise his or her tongue since it should be getting more than enough exercise every day in just talking alone. As easy as this is to understand, it misses the fact that talking (and using the tongue when eating) only employ the tongue in a limited range of motions compared to the ones described below. Quite frankly, while the tongue is used a great deal by some people, one rarely gets this little muscle tired. It is never really "exercised" in the strict meaning of that word. Therefore, exercising it for the purpose of really getting the circulation going is the point of the immediate discussion. **Tongue exercises improve blood flow and improve functions of internal organs through meridians.**

The Exercises

Although you can easily come up with a variety of 'athletic events' for your tongue, I will mention a few that are simple and easily done.

3. Stick your tongue straight out as far as you can and then curl it inwards towards the back of your mouth as far as you can. Repeat until the tongue is tired.
4. Move your tongue slowly in a circular motion in front of your teeth while reaching as far as you can with your tongue. Do 3 - 5 circles clockwise and then repeat in a counterclockwise direction. Repeat until tongue is tired.
5. Stick your tongue straight out of your mouth as far as you can and move it rapidly side to side. Repeat until tongue is tired.

Caution. These exercises can be done safely by most anyone. However, if you have a pre-existing medical condition with the tongue or the mouth area, you should consult your primary health care professional before attempting these exercises. Persons with a history of involuntarily swallowing their tongues should not do these exercises. Also, since these can be easily done in the car while driving, please make sure that your performance of these exercises does not constitute "distracted driving." You may also want to make sure that these exercises do not become a *performance* for other drivers.

Conclusion: *The tongue is the beginning of the digestive system. Through nerves and vessels it is connected with all the digestive organs. The tongue, esophagus, stomach, small intestine, and colon all make up one continuous chain. Therefore, by cleansing the tongue and doing exercises for the tongue, we activate the whole digestive system, improve its function, and increase digestion.*

"... My 9-year-old son suffered from enlarged tonsils, which were supposed to be surgically removed. I knew that I do not want him to go through this, but didn't even realize how important tonsils are for his immune system. Dr. Koyfman explained to me the importance of healthy tonsils and gave his recommendations on how to help my boy. After a very short period of time his tonsils went back to normal size and the pain was gone. It was so simple to follow his advice and instructions, even my 9-year-old had no problems doing so. Now my whole family consults with Dr. Koyfman regarding their health and well-being..."

Mrs. Robinson

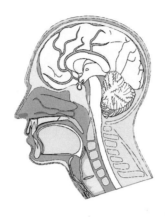

Throat

Throat is not only a pathway for food and air, but together with tonsils– it is a barrier designated to catch bacteria and infections, which get in the mouth from unclean foods, beverages and infected gums. Tonsils and throat can also be infected by air that does not go through proper cleansing treatment in the nose and sinuses. For example if breathing occurs directly through the mouth (especially if the air is cold) due to the nose congestion.

Tonsils do not only catch the bacteria, but also produce necessary agents to kill it. However, when tonsils become filled with bacteria, they are not able to lead that fight on their own. So when tonsils loose the ability to control spreading of infection, the body signals it by causing pain in the throat or "soar throat". That is the time, when it is almost too late, but still possible to stop spreading of infection and illness deep into the body. However, if you ignore that signal (your body's scream for help) the illness penetrates deeper in the body and can cause more serious consequences, such as bronchitis, cough, cold, flue, angina, digestive problems, etc.

Unique recipes and methods described in this chapter, will help you not only prevent throat and tonsil disorders, but also prevent more serious problems, illnesses, colds and stomach disease.

Some Problems with the Throat

Throat Inflammation

A sore, red throat, along with an elevated temperature points to the presence of an infection. Redness in the throat can also be caused by flu or cold.

Laryngitis

In its acute form laryngitis is a bacterial or viral infection of the larynx (voice box). It can make swallowing difficult, and one can temporarily lose the ability to speak. This more serious form can develop into tonsillitis, bronchitis, pneumonia or flu. In its lesser form (chronic laryngitis) difficulty in swallowing and speaking may be symptoms.

Tonsillitis

The tonsils are a pair of glands located on both sides of the throat. These two small glands are designed to trap bacteria and viruses before they get any further into the body. They also produce antibodies to fight infections. When infections overwhelm the tonsils they increase in size, their surface becomes covered with pus, and they become inflamed. The throat becomes sore and fever may develop. When this happens frequently, it can lead to a chronic enlargement of the tonsils. Sometimes infection from tonsils can spread to the middle ear through the Eustachian channel. I know from experience that **if you have a sore throat and don't take care of it right away the infection can quickly spread to the bronchi, causing coughing and bronchitis.**

Techniques for Keeping Your Throat Clean and Healthy

Rinsing

You can rinse your throat with a wide variety of different mixtures. For example:

1. One teaspoon of *sea salt* to one cup of warm water.
2. One teaspoon of *baking soda* to one cup of warm water.
3. One teaspoon of *apple cider vinegar* to one cup of water.
4. *Garlic* rinse. Mash 1 - 2 cloves of garlic and put in a cup of hot water. When the water cools down, strain and use it to rinse your throat.
5. *Propolis mixture* rinse. Add 10-15 drops of propolis extract to one cup of warm water. Mix thoroughly and rinse your throat. Propolis is sold in Health Stores.
6. You can also use *extracts from herbs* such as chamomile, sage, etc.
7. *Lemon juice* can be very good for throat rinses. You can dilute it with water or just use as it is.

Rinsing Technique

Take some of the rinsing mixture in your mouth, tilt your head backward, inhale some air through your nose and slowly exhale it through the mouth making a "grrrrrr" sound. When you run out of air, inhale some more through the nose and repeat the procedure. This rinsing technique helps in pulling mucus from tonsils. As a preventive measure you can rinse your throat every morning when brushing your teeth. If your throat is inflamed you can do rinses every two hours or even every hour.

Lion Pose

Sit on a chair, or on the floor with legs under you and your palms on knees. (You can also do this exercise standing up.) Inhale deeply, and then slowly exhale from the mouth while simultaneously sticking your tongue out as far as possible and keeping the muscles of the root of the tongue and of the throat tense. Hold your breath for a few seconds maintaining medium tension. Relax throat muscles at the same time inhaling more air through your nose. Repeat 3-5 times. Rinse your throat with any of the previously mentioned mixtures or just with clean water.

Therapeutic Effects

When muscles of the throat, face and tongue are tense blood is pushed out of this area by the pressure from the muscles. When muscles relax the blood comes back as a fast moving stream (because tension creates contraction and relaxation releases the "spring"). The stream of blood breaks down blockages and washes out toxins accumulated in that area. Removal of blockages and wastes activates circulation in the area. Rinsing after doing a Lion Pose removes toxins/mucus, which were on the surface and those, which came from the inside of tissues.

During inflammation of the throat you can repeat Lion Pose 5-7 or more times.

Throat Massage

The self-massage of the throat also works on improving circulation in this part of the body, and in washing out toxins.

Massage Technique

This technique can be performed while you stand, sit or lay on your back. This massage can be done with your palms, fingers or the back of your hands. Also, you can use circular, up-and-down, and spreading motions to effect the massage. Under all circumstances, use light to moderate pressure when massaging the throat. Choose your motions based on whatever works best for you. Follow your intuition. Use some oil or lotion. Massage for 2-3 minutes.

Exercises

Exercises for the neck have the same goal as other exercises: to activate blood flow, remove toxins, improve flexibility, and reduce stress of muscles. (You can find descriptions of these exercises in my book, *Unique Method of Colon Rejuvenation*). Your morning routine could include the yoga exercise called "Fish." It is very good for activating blood flow in the throat.

The exercises, massages, and poses described here not only improve blood circulation in the throat, but also activate circulation and cleanse the thyroid and parathyroid glands. This plays a major role in maintaining good health.

Natural Antibiotic for the Throat

Again **garlic** in its raw, natural state comes to the rescue. Whenever you get a sore throat, or throat infection, use fresh raw garlic to kill the infection. To do this, peel one clove of garlic, and then put it in your mouth on your tongue. Suck on the clove of garlic as if it's a candy and swallow the saliva. (Do NOT chew it unless you have done that before and are up to it.) Keep it in your mouth as long as you can (hopefully 10 - 20 minutes). This procedure can be repeated 3 - 5 times during the day. The pain in your throat should disappear within one day. During cold and flu season this procedure can be performed as a preventive measure.

Propolis has the same wonderful characteristic as garlic. (Propolis is a substance made by honeybees from plant resins.) Take a little piece of it and put in your mouth for a short period of time. (It is safe to chew propolis.) Swallow the saliva. Both propolis and garlic help in cleansing of throat, gums and blood. If you find propolis in liquid form, then use 10 to 20 drops of this extract in 6 to 8 oz. warm water or warm camomile tea to rinse your mouth and throat. **This rinsing will kill infection in the throat, tonsils, and gums.**

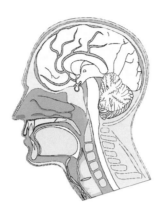

Nose and Sinuses

Nose passages and sinuses are not only pathways for air, but are also barriers (filters) designated to stop and not allow entering of bad bacteria, infection, dust and other harmful particles present in the air. This filtration is necessary in order to not allow infection and "dirt" to get into the bronchi and lungs, and to also prevent illnesses of these organs (cough, bronchitis, pneumonia, colds and flue).

To not allow spreading of infection deep in the system and prevent serious illnesses– it is necessary to always keep nose passages and sinuses clean, healthy and clear. If both nose and sinuses are blocked with toxic mucus and other impurities, they do not only loose the ability to cleanse the air, warm-up it up and catch infection, but become ill as well. This process is often caused by overcooling, exhaustion, stress, foods containing mucus forming products, etc.

Learn in this chapter how to quickly help your-selves and relatives with colds and chronic illnesses of the nose and sinuses. Most importantly, learn how to prevent those illnesses with simple methods and always available to you ingredients.

Some Problems with the Nose and Sinuses

Because of all of these diverse connections it is easy to understand how infections can spread throughout the head.

Chronic Rhinitis

This nasal disease can be caused by allergies, sinusitis, or the prolonged use of aerosols and medicines. If caused by allergies, the symptoms would include the secretion of a lot of nasal fluids punctuated by plenty of sneezing. If caused by sinusitis, nasal secretions would contain mucus and puss.

Pollen Allergy

Allergies afflict the human nose and respiratory system to such a large extent that entire industries are built around relieving the symptoms. Allergies that torment the nose are often caused by one or more plants, and are more common in the spring and summer time. Major symptoms are sneezing, teary eyes, and a runny nose. Some people develop a weak form of asthma along with a feeling tension in the chest.

Sinusitis

This is inflammation of the sinus cavities. It usually starts after a cold, and can result in headaches, fever, and nasal secretions containing blood. Skin, which covers the inflamed cavities, is always very sensitive.

How to Keep Your Nose and Sinuses Clean and Healthy

Keeping the nose passages and sinuses clean improves the quality of air inhaled, ease in breathing, oxygenation of cells in the whole system and particularly the in brain. It prevents colds, infections, and allergies.

Start by maintaining a healthy lifestyle. By that I mean a conscious effort to help your body cleanse itself of toxicity; provide your body with a sufficient amount of natural vitamins, minerals, proteins, carbohydrates, etc.; strengthening internal organs and muscles through special exercises; give your lungs a chance to receive clean air as described earlier; follow healthy daily biorhythms of sleep, eating and working; and give your body a chance to rest and relax as appropriate.

A healthy lifestyle also includes reducing, avoiding or eliminating anything that damages the body. This includes such actions and conditions as stress, overeating, overheating, not getting enough sleep, exhaustion, smoking, alcohol, medicines, junk food, etc. It's understandable that in reality we cannot completely eliminate all damaging events. But if we do whatever we reasonably can to counteract these events we can help our body come out on top in this struggle.

51

If you have never done any cleansings start with a series of colonics, followed by a liver cleanse and then other cleansing procedures as called for by your personal circumstances. These cleansings will sharply decrease the level of toxic mucus and other substances in your body, and will strengthen your immune system. Now, to maintain it, you need to perform every day one or more of the cleansing procedures described below.

Nose and Sinuses Rinse Using Your Hands

This procedure is very simple to perform, **does not take any significant time,** and is easily done with any other water-related activities such as washing your hands or face, or taking a shower. It can be easily done a few times a day. Why so often you might ask?

In the morning, when we wake up, the internal surface of the nose is dried as a result of heaters or air conditioners, and the fact that we can not drink water as we sleep in order to rehydrate. The internal surface of the nose is also begrimed by the fact that the tiny hairs it bears have been filtering your breathing air all night, and you have not been able to get rid of the accumulated waste during that rest. The morning rinse helps to get rid of those.

During the day we can at least take some reasonable actions to cleanse these areas as they gather dust, pollen and bacteria inside the nose. Afternoon rinses help to wash out these collections from nose and sinuses. In the evenings, before going to bed, we can also easily perform this procedure and go to sleep with a clean nose, which will help assure light and easy breathing all night.

The procedure described below is also recommended immediately after you feel accumulation of mucus in your

nose or throat, or reaction from allergies. At that time you should rinse your nose and throat a few times and you will feel relief right away. If you only blow out your nose without using the technique below it does not allow you to quickly get rid of mucus and irritation.

Technique for Nose and Sinus Cleansing

First, while standing in front of a sink or while in the shower, form a "cup" with one hand by putting your fingers together with that hand palm up. Next fill this "cup" with room temperature water. (Since you will not be drinking this water, tap water is acceptable if it is clean and filtered.) Bend your body at the waist, and insert your nose completely in the water. With a short inhalation, suck the water up into your nose being careful not to pull it in too deeply. After you have pulled some water into your nose, move your hand away. Quickly close one nostril completely by pressing against one side of your nose with your fingers. Immediately do 1 - 2 sharp exhalations through the other (open) nostril to blow waste from that nostril. Then cover up the other nostril and exhale sharply through it. Put more water in your hand again and repeat pulling in water and blowing out your nose. You can perform this cycle 3 - 5 times, until your nasal passages are clean.

How You Can Check If Your Nasal Passages Are Clean

1. Use your index finger to press one nostril closed. Then inhale through the other nostril. You can feel whether or

not this other nostril is open. If you can inhale easily, it is open. If you find it difficult to inhale, then that nostril is blocked. Release your finger from the closed nostril, then repeat by closing off the nostril you already tested in order to test the other nostril.

2. Carefully insert the pinkies of each hand into your nostrils as far as you can without damaging sensitive nasal tissues. (Nails should be cut short and fingers clean). In this manner you can feel if there is any mucus or dried up matter left in your nose. If the internal surface is still not clean you can repeat this procedure or try others described below.

Cleansing the Nose and Sinuses through Sneezing

Sometimes after you have pulled water into your nose and then blown air through the nasal passages to eliminate water, mucus, and bacteria, there is water which remains in the nasal passages and creates sneezing.

Nature uses sneezing during illnesses, colds, flu, allergies, etc., to cleanse the sinuses, nasal passages, and the entire pulmonary system and its organs. Sneezing begins with irritation in the nasal passages when you have a runny nose. At this time you automatically take a deep inhalation of breath, making the first sound, "Ah . . ." During this inhalation your chest and lungs expand like a balloon, and then a strong exhalation squeezes air out through the nose and mouth with the second sound, "Choo!" With the air, our body pushes out toxic mucus and bacteria, not only from the nasal passages but also from the lungs, bronchi, throat, and eyes. Our eyes become wet with tears and the tears cleanse the eyes.

When we get ill our system repeats this process so many times we begin to feel uncomfortable from it. But we don't need to wait until we get ill to start sneezing and help our system to get rid of mucus and infection. We can create sneezing artificially when we pull water into the nose to cleanse our sinuses. If some water stays in the nose, it will create irritation and cleansing sneezing. It won't happen every time, but when it happens, you can consciously help your system to eliminate more mucus and toxins. In the moment when you start feeling the sneeze you can consciously deepen the automatic inhalation, and after that you can consciously increase the speed and strength of the exhalation. This will help to eliminate a large amount of mucus and bacteria, which accumulate in the pulmonary system.

You can also create sneezing when you do the internal nose massage with soap.

Sneezing can sometimes happen 2-3 times in a row. After the sneezing, you need to clean your nose with water again. Also, clean your throat through gargling because sneezing draws mucus from the tonsils and other tissue, and you may feel that your throat and mouth are filled with mucus.

Conscious sneezing also improves circulation in the abdominal organs, chest, and head, including the blood vessels in the brain (through the vibration caused by the sharp shaking of the head).

The Neti Pot Nasal Rinse

This procedure is designed for deeper rinsing of the nasal and sinus passages.

1. **It helps to wash out harder-to-remove accumulations** from the sinuses and nose when a standard rinse is not sufficient.
2. **It also kills and washes out infection.** It can be done 1 - 2 times per week for mild symptoms; or if you have a bad cold, stuffy nose or headache it can be done 3 - 5 times a day until you get satisfactory results.
3. **It activates the trigeminal nerve,** which connects to the ears, the eyes, and the sinuses, and may help to improve vision and hearing.

Equipment and Materials

Before you begin, assemble all of the materials that you will need in the area where you will be doing the procedure. Take 16 fluid ounces of clean water and add 1 teaspoon of sea salt and 5 drops of iodine. Mix well. (Omit the iodine if you are allergic to iodine.)

You will also need a specialized Neti pot that is typically found in health-oriented stores. This is a kind of teapot with a very narrow spout that can fit into one nostril. (If you can't find one of these Neti pots you can use a regular, small teapot by covering its opening with a rubber stopper. This rubber stopper should have an external diameter of approximately 1/8th inch to 1/4th inch or 3 - 5 mm diameter, and should have a small opening in it. Avoid any teapot with an aluminum interior.)

Procedure

Put clean water in a saucepan, and heat it to a temperature slightly higher than your own normal body temperature. If you are measuring the water temperature with a thermometer it should be approximately 100° to 104° F, or 38° to 40° C. Remember that these numbers are not magic, and that what really counts is for you to find (by experience) a water temperature that is warm enough to loosen encrusted or very viscous waste material while feeling comfortable. (Natural heat is better than heating the water in a microwave.) Put the clean, warm water in a Neti pot.

Stand over a sink and hold the Neti pot in your hand. Make sure you are comfortable. *Carefully* insert the spout of the Neti pot into one of your nostrils, and tilt your head in the opposite direction by about 45 degrees. Slightly bend your body forward. You can use your other hand to hold yourself steady. Open your mouth and breath through your mouth during this procedure.

Now, tilt the Neti pot so that the water starts running into your nose. The warm, salty water will go through your nasal passages into your nasal cavities where it will soften accumulated waste matter and help it to break free. When this procedure is performed correctly the water will exit through the other nostril carrying the waste with it. If you are not holding your head at the proper angle a little bit of water can flow into your mouth. Spit it out. Do not swallow it because it contains waste products.

After all of the water is gone, close the nostril in which the water was coming in and do a few short exhalations through the opposite nostril. Then close the other nostril and do a few short exhalations through it. **Caution:** The force of exhalation should be moderate in strength and short in duration.

Exhalations that are too strong or long can send the water into ears through the Eustachian tubes. There is no advantage in this. Generally speaking, **never blow out your nose with too much force.**

Repeat the procedure for the other nostril. Remember that some water may be left in your nasal passages after performing this procedure, but it will come out on its own. That is normal. **Caution:** If it is cold outside you should stay indoors where it is warm for at least one hour. Otherwise, the water still left in your nasal passages can become cold and cause health problems.

For Hard-to-Convince Noses

If your nose and/or nasal passages are *really* stuffed-up with a lot of encrusted or hard to remove waste matter, then there is a way to soften this material prior to performing the Neti Pot Nasal Rinse described above. To accomplish this you can use the steam from cooked potatoes.

Boil unpeeled potatoes in a covered pot. While the potatoes are boiling take two chairs and arrange them so that they are facing each other. Put a thick towel (beach towel) folded up in one chair to protect the chair from heat. You will be sitting in the other chair. Put a medium size towel on the back of the chair you will be sitting in so that it will be ready for you.

After boiling the potatoes, put the *covered* pot (with the potatoes still in the pot) in the chair with the folded up towel, and take a seat in the other chair. Drape the second towel over your head so that it forms a hood over your head. Bend over the pot and gradually remove the cover from it, slowly enough so as not to let so much steam escape as to burn your face. As the steam comes up, breathe in the steam slowly and deeply through your nose. Exhale through your mouth.

Be careful when you first do this technique not to get too close to the steam so that it is not uncomfortably hot for you. Start a little further away from the steam at first, and then determine the best distance by experimenting. Sit over the steam in this manner for 10 - 15 minutes, and then rinse your nose and sinus passages using the Neti Pot Nasal Cleanse.

The Grand Mariner Rinse

Sucking up water with your nose has the same basic therapeutic effects as the Neti Pot Nasal Rinse technique, but with one significant difference. This procedure requires greater effort to master. If you choose to learn it, you will also become more versatile in the other methods of nasal and sinus cleansing. One other characteristic of this method of cleansing is that by sucking up water with your nose you are also exercising "the sucking muscles" which will result in a more active cleansing of the pathway connecting nose and mouth.

Technique

To perform this procedure you will need a wide container capable of holding approximately one quart (a little more than one liter) of liquid. Prepare this amount of clean water by heating it to a little warmer than body temperature. (See directions for water temperature in the Neti Pot Nasal Rinse above.) Put all of the water in your container, and add two teaspoons of sea salt. Mix well.

Stand over a sink holding the container with both hands and submerge your nose into the salty water. Exhale through your mouth, and start pulling in water through both nostrils by slowly inhaling the salty water. The water will begin to enter your mouth, which should be closed. When your mouth becomes full of water, spit it out into the sink. Then, without taking your nose out of the water, inhale a breath of air and exhale that air through your mouth. Repeat the procedure of pulling water through both nostrils again until you become tired or you run out of water.

After you have finished, close one nostril and do a few short exhalations through it. Then close the other nostril and do a few short exhalations through that one. **To repeat:** The force of exhalation should be moderate in strength and short in duration. Exhalations that are too strong or long can send the water into ears through the Eustachian tubes. There is no advantage in this. Generally speaking, never blow out your nose with too much force.

After this procedure there may be a little left over water in your nasal and sinus passages. This water may drip out for a short period of time. This is normal. To speed up the process of removing water bend your body forward and move your head from side to side a few times.

Remember, if it is cold outside you should stay indoors where it is warm for at least one hour. Otherwise, any water still left in your nasal passages can become cold and cause health problems.

For blowing sinuses out with air see page 22 of my book, *Unique Method of Colon Rejuvenation.*

External Nose Massage

The value of massaging the outside of your nose is that this procedure activates the flow of blood, warms up the nose tissues and any thickened mucus, and helps to ease and deepen breathing.

Technique

1. Use both of your index fingers and start rubbing the external surface of your nose beginning from the top and moving towards the tip of your nose. Use either up and down, or circular motions. Repeat until your nose feels warmed up.
2. Slightly bend both thumbs and rub the sides of your nose until it feels warmed up.

Internal Nose Massage

This technique helps to wash out mucus and dirt stuck to the walls of the nose, and helps to widen nasal passages which makes breathing easier. Internal nose massage with natural soap kills bacteria and viruses found there. Although we cannot reach sinuses with our fingers the smell of the soap gets in there and kills the bacteria. Be sure you understand that this is not a method of removing waste. It is a massage technique.

Technique

1. Make sure your fingernails are cut short, and are not sharp. Also, make sure your fingers are thoroughly clean, especially under the fingernails
2. Wet your pinky fingers with water. Carefully put your fingers into your nostrils and slowly make your way upward as far as possible. Then turn them a few degrees

and take them out. Wash your fingers carefully and repeat the procedure a few more times.

3. Do the same thing but instead of wetting your fingers with water use some natural soap.

Then wash off your fingers and rinse your nose with water by any of the above-described methods.

Inhaling Garlic Vapor

Garlic is a natural antibiotic. Its vapors contain natural substances which are capable of killing infections. The vapors are effective not only in sinuses, but also in bronchi and lungs. The procedure of inhaling garlic vapors can be used when you have a cold, or as a preventive measure during cold and flu season.

Cut fresh, raw garlic into small pieces and put the pieces on a small plate. Leave the plate near your bed when you are sleeping. You will inhale garlic vapors during your sleep. If the smell is too strong move the plate a little further away from you. This procedure is especially useful for small children who cannot yet do nasal/sinus rinses.

Besides using garlic, some of the other things available for children are different kinds of natural nose drops, such as onion juice diluted with water, beet juice, etc.

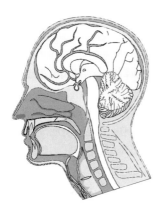

Ears

Understanding the Human Ear

The human ear is divided into three basic parts: the outer, the middle and inner ear. The outer and middle ear collect sound waves which they pass to the ear drum (in the inner ear) through the ear canal. When sound waves hit the eardrum it starts to vibrate which enables us to hear. The middle ear is connected to the throat by the Eustachian tubes. If one or both of Eustachian tubes becomes blocked as a result of inflammation the eardrum loses its ability to freely vibrate, and hearing temporarily becomes impaired.

63

Some Problems with the Ear

A Pain in the Ear

Ear pain can be caused by several different situations, such as a large accumulation of wax, the intrusion of a foreign object into the ear canal, exposure to very loud sounds, or by a reaction to chemicals such as hair spray, shampoo or chlorine from a swimming pool. But in most cases ear pain is caused by an infection of the outer or middle ear. Pain in the ear can also develop if water gets into it during swimming, especially if there is a lot of wax accumulated there. (Excess ear wax can be the result of too much mucus accumulating in the head area.)

Phantom Ear Noise

Depending on age and/or heredity, some people experience hearing loss and some begin hearing noises which only they can hear. This particular malady is called Tinnitus. Noises can range from high pitched sounds to low grade hums. Some simply describe the sound as Grand Central Station because of the diversity of noise and the loud volume. For some sufferers, the duration of the sound is brief, while for others it almost never stops.

Abscesses

Skin abscess around the ears or even in the ear canal usually lead to irritation and scratching. This in turn can lead to these areas becoming infected.

What You Can Do to Protect the Health of Your Ears

With the exception of a physical injury to the ears by some trauma, **most ear problems are the result of personal body pollution or toxicity, especially toxic mucus in the area of the head. Therefore, the cure and prevention of these problems starts with cleansing the body, and with maintaining a daily healthy life style.** If the problem is old and does not go away fast enough it is best to attack it with both traditional and alternative methods. But if you regularly cleanse your body, eat a healthy diet, exercise and take care of your body's organs and systems, you can eliminate most problems described above.

Ear Hygiene

Cleansing the outer part of the ear and ear canal (middle ear) should be achieved during daily face rinses and during daily showers. The technique is simple and basic. After putting some natural soap on your index and middle fingers, clean the external part of your ears, the beginning of the ear canal and behind the ears. Wash off the soap from both ears. (It is best if your shower has a water filter. These will eliminate chlorine, which can irritate ears and eyes.) After your shower is over, a little bit of water is usually left in the ears, and ear wax has become soft. To get rid of the water and any excessive ear wax use "Q-tips" after each shower. Be very careful when using those so you don't damage your eardrums. The cleanliness of internal parts of the ears is maintained by cleansing the large intestine, small intestine, liver and nose (as described above). **If you take care of your nose and sinuses then the inner ear should stay clean.**

Ear Massage

The surface of the outer ear contains a number of acupuncture points connected to the internal organs through meridians. Massage of the ears stimulates the blood flow in the ears (to improve their functioning) and stimulates the internal organs gently stimulating them as well.

Ear Massage Technique

Massage is performed using the thumb and it opposing index finger. Gently grab your ears so that your thumbs are touching them from the back and your index fingers are touching them from the front. Apply light pressure with your fingers, and use a rubbing motion to move from the bottom of the ear to the top. You can change the position of your fingers to achieve the most comfortable position. Rub and gently pull on the ears until you feel that they are warm. Then using your index finger trace the folds of the ears and massage the ear canal. Then extend the middle and index finger and bend your ears to form a V-shape. Press index fingers against the front of the ear and middle fingers against the back and make rubbing back and forth motions to warm up these areas. Then press the palms of your hands against your ears and grab the back of your ears with your fingers. Make a few rubbing and stretching motions and end the massage.

Exercises to Improve Hearing

Stand straight up with your hands at your sides. Breathe in calmly and slowly through your nose, and breathe out in the same manner. Use your thumbs to close off the ear canals. Use your middle fingers to close of your nasal passages by pressing on the sides of the nose. Put your lips together as if you were whistling and take a fast, sharp and short breath filling up your mouth with air. Lower your head and rest your chin on your chest. Close your eyes and put your index fingers on your eyelids without using any pressure. Hold your breath in this position until you experience the first signs of discomfort. To exit this pose: raise your head to the starting position, leaving your hands in the same position, move your index fingers from your eye lids, open your eyes, then move your fingers from your nose. After that, calmly and slowly breathe out through your nose, move your thumbs from your ears and put your arms in the starting position and inhale in a regular way. This exercise is performed one time per day. **Besides helping to improve your hearing, this exercise has a positive effect on your eyes and helps with sinusitis.**

Some More Exercises

All yoga exercises where the head is positioned below the body also improve circulation in all organs of the head, including ears, and help in improving hearing. Some exercises of this type are described in my book, *Unique Method of Colon Regeneration.* These include using a "slant board." These exercises also benefit the functioning of the colon.

What to Do If You Have Ear Pain

As mentioned earlier, ear pain can be caused by an accumulation of dirt or by an infection of the middle ear. Therefore, the goal is to clean one's ears and kill any infections.

To clean the ear of dirt and toxicity you can use a little bulb syringe, which can be purchased in any drug store. Fill it up with clean, warm water, and **using light pressure**, spray some water in the ear. While doing this, tilt your head to the side so that the "bad ear" is higher. (This procedure should be performed over the sink.) If one rinse is not enough, you can repeat this procedure a few more times. Then, soak up the rest of the water with cotton balls.

Then, take a fresh, raw onion, and juice it. Strain the juice. (Onion is a natural antibiotic and its juices can kill many kinds of infections.) Put the onion juice in a dropper, lay on a bed and drop 3 - 5 drops of the onion juice into your ear. (Its better if someone else does it for you.) Cover that ear canal with a cotton ball to retain warmth and lay down for 20 minutes. Then, clean the ear of onion juice with a cotton ball and repeat this procedure using the same dosage. Lay down for another 20 minutes. If pain does not stop you can repeat the procedure one more time. Most of the time this should be enough to completely stop, or at least to lower, the pain. If necessary, you can repeat this procedure 2 - 3 days in a row.

Improving Your Hearing Using Concentration

In today's world we are barraged with information, much of it in an auditory form. This includes radio, television, conversations both by telephone and face-to-face, etc. We are also inundated by a wide variety of noises not meant to communicate anything in particular. All of this works together to desensitize our hearing just as a self-protection mechanism from information and auditory overload. Every once in a while we should "recalibrate" our hearing with exercises designed to increase our hearing sensitivity. Fortunately, there is a simple and pleasant exercise for doing just that. This "exercise" can really be considered a form of meditation.

Sit in a comfortable chair or lay down on a bed, close your eyes, and relax your muscles. Start listening to the surrounding sounds. At first, you will only hear louder sounds, but then you should be able to distinguish the quieter sounds. For example, at first you may hear the sound of passing cars or airplanes, dogs barking, etc. But as you concentrate more you will also hear less discernable sounds such as birds chirping, the wind, small noises inside your home, etc. Most importantly relax when you're listening, try to hear and distinguish all of the sounds. Stay in this position for 10 - 15 minutes. As you search the world around you with your ears you will begin to realize how much you may have missed. **This exercise not only increases the sensitivity of your hearing, but will also allow you to have some rest and to boost up your energy.** Feel free to do this exercise as often as you like.

Finally Free!

All my life I've suffered from constipation. At age 20, I started totally falling apart. I had constant flues, colds, sinus infections and soar throats. My nose was constantly clogged and I forgot what it's like to breath through my nose. Medical doctors kept putting me on antibiotics, which were not helping my symptoms, but did a great job on ruining my digestive system completely. I was on laxatives everyday; started getting yeast infections; had constant heartburn. Eventually I got a soar throat which lasted for over two months and didn't seem to be going anywhere. I couldn't speak, eat and every time I would swallow, it felt like knives were passing through. Doctors kept changing their antibiotic prescription and finally gave up saying that they don't know what to do. My friend saw Dr. Koyfman's article in the newspaper and told me to try it. At that point I was ready for anything! Not knowing where I was going or what would be done, I ended up at the Koyfman Whole Body Cleansing. During my first session I had nothing but mucus coming out of my body and that same evening, my soar throat was gone. It took a few more procedures before my sinuses cleared up and a few more to get my digestion back to normal. I am finally free off constipation and suffocation. I am able to breath normally. I changed my whole life style and enjoy it very much. I feel very lucky that I actually got sick so early in life and was able to find Dr. Koyfman who set me in the right direction for the future.

Helen Rybak, Atlanta, GA

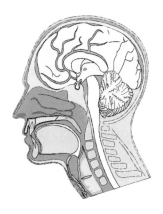

Salivary Glands

Cleansing of the Salivary Glands

The human mouth has six salivary glands: four under the tongue and two in front of the ears, one on each side. The main function of salivary glands is to produce and secrete saliva, which flow through many canals into the mouth. There saliva mixes up with food, which should have been thoroughly chewed.

The more the food is chewed the better it will mix with saliva. This is important because **saliva is the first stage of digesting food.** Saliva also wets the food and makes swallowing easier. Some substances found in saliva have bacteriocidal functions. Some substances which stop the development of AIDS are thought to be in saliva. Saliva is slightly basic with a pH ranging from 7.4 to 8.0. Basic pH neutralizes the actions of acids preventing degradation of teeth.

Proper Chewing and Blood Cleansing

All fluids of the body - stomach juices, saliva, lymph, tissue fluids, etc. - are made from blood. During chewing the amount of blood flowing thru salivary glands increases 3 - 4 times. **In fact, the salivary glands make saliva from blood. When this happens the salivary glands work like filters, removing harmful products of metabolism from the blood. That's why if you chew your food using the method described in my book** *Deep Internal Body Cleansing* **you can maintain a good level of blood cleanliness,** if of course you don't poison it with bad food products.

The concept of cleansing blood while chewing explains why if you don't feel good during a fast it is usually enough to chew on some vegetable or fruit, without swallowing it, to feel relief. Not feeling good during a fast is due to the fact that blood becomes saturated with toxic substances which get released from cells throughout the body.

From everything described above we can see how important salivary glands are in digestion, prevention of teeth decay and in blood filtering. Therefore, it's necessary to keep them healthy.

Principles of Maintaining the Health of the Salivary Glands

1. **The process of chewing,** if done correctly, is a great way to stimulate salivary glands.
2. **Neck exercises** described in my book *Unique Method of Colon Rejuvenation* are also good for stimulating blood flow in salivary glands.
3. **Direct massage of the neck and salivary glands** improves blood circulation, and helps in cleansing of salivary glands. The areas to massage are the front part of the neck, under the jaw and in front of the ears. Lightly rub these areas with your fingers or palms until you feel warmth.
4. **Consuming sufficient amount of liquids,** clean water, herb tea and fresh juices during the day also helps in cleansing and maintaining healthy salivary glands.
5. Occasional breaks from "work" are also beneficial for the functions of salivary glands. These breaks are **24 to 36 hour fasts consuming only water, herbal teas or juices diluted with water.** These fasts can be done once a week or once every two weeks depending on individual circumstances. During the fast you consume large amounts of liquids, which help to cleanse salivary glands without stressing them so that they get their "rest."

Pollen Season

Since coming to the center I have felt increased energy and better body awareness. For the first time in over 15 years this pollen season had no effect on me. Usually, I struggle with sinuses and colds all during pollen season, but this year I had none of these symptoms. I have noticed many other effects and health benefits as well. I have recommended these treatments to many other people who noticed similar benefits.

-- Tim R.--

Rabbits and Snails

When I first came here, my eyes looked as red as rabbit's eyes and I moved as fast as a snail. I had been diagnosed with Chronic Fatigue Syndrome and I was sick all the time. I was feeling extremely depressed and this place was my last hope, because there is no allopathic cure for this disease. A year later, I can say I the right thing about following Dr. Koyfman's treatments and life style suggestions. Now I don't stay in bed all the time and I have wonderful plans for the future. I exercise, I sleep well, and I lost weight. I am a happy camper!

--Teresa Emmers--

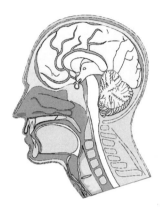

Eyes

Some Diseases of the Eye

One of the big differences between alternative medicine and traditional medicine is that alternative medicine is much more focused on prevention, whereas traditional medicine is more focused on cure. Because of this the main goal of the methods in this book is prevention.

If you do have a problem in the beginning stages, you may find the techniques here useful, but if you have a disease that has been going on for a while, don't waste any time. Go directly to a traditional doctor to be diagnosed and then decide if you want to treat it using traditional or alternative medicine. I think that **with any serious disease the best solution is a combination of traditional and alternative methods.**

Conjunctivitis

Conjunctivitis is an inflammation of the mucus membrane which covers the insides of the eyelid and part of the eyeball. The conjunctivitis discharge from the eye makes eyelids stick together. Conjunctivitis is contagious and can spread from one eye to the other.

Inflammation of Eyelids

Redness of the eyelids is most commonly connected with abscess on some part of the body, usually on the skull under the hair. Eyelids can become irritated and scabby.

Irritation and Tearing

These symptoms are usually caused by allergies. If you know what you are allergic to the best approach is distance from the allergic substance. If that is not possible or practical, then cleansing is vital.

Eye Strain

People who read a lot or who spend a lot of time in front of the computer, often develop eyestrain. Symptoms are pain in the eyes and headaches.

Cherry Eye

Cherry eye is a small abscess on one or more eyelids. The first sign of the development of abscess is irritation of eyelids. Then it becomes red, painful, and inflamed.

Eye Diagnostics

Examining your eyes can often provide valuable clues to health conditions throughout the body.

For example: **excessive blinking** points to nervousness, anxiety and fear.

Dropped eyelids point to a feeling of insecurity, loss of confidence and fear.

If the eyes bulge out it means that there is some disruption in the work of thyroid gland.

If the conjunctive is pale it means that you might be anemic.

If the conjunctive is yellow there is a problem with the liver.

A small iris points to weakness of in the joints.

If there is a white circle around the iris it means that there is an excess of sugar or salt. In middle-aged people this could be a symptom of stress.

If the circles are really pronounced and really white it means that the joints are very fragile, they could be easily fractured. Pain and arthritis are possible. This would point to a calcium deficiency in the body.

Dark brown spots on the iris mean that intestine is not absorbing iron properly.

Even without knowing all of this, if you look into a person's eyes *you can intuitively feel his weaknesses and strengths,* if he is honest or if he is healthy. There is a *special spark in the eyes* of people who are involved, healthy and clean especially *after the fast.* People who are "enlightened" have the most interesting eyes.

How to Daily Maintain the Health of the Eyes

Eighty-three percent of the information received by the brain comes through the eyes. Eyes are our windows to the outside world and the cleaner these windows the more realistically we see our surroundings.

Through nerves, the eyes are connected to the brain. Eye massage and eye exercises not only improve the vision, but also, through the nerves, affect brain function and improve it. Regularly doing eye exercise and eye massage improves circulation in the eyes which leads to their better nourishment and cleansing. This massage and exercise prevents eye illnesses and headaches, helps to normalize blood pressure, and increases energy and endurance.

Massage of the Eyes

Sit in a comfortable position with your back straight. Breathe freely and close your eyes. Put the palms of your hands on your eyes. With *light* circular motions massage the eyeballs for 10-20 seconds. Then slowly move your palms, blink a few times and relax your eyes. Perform these exercises anytime you feel that your eyes are tired.

Exercise 1

Sit in a comfortable position with your back straight. Breathe freely and close your eyes. Keep your head still. Slowly look to the left as far as you can and focus for a second. Then slowly move your eyes and look to the right. Focus for a second. Repeat 5 - 10 times on each side. Close your eyes and relax for a few seconds. Open your eyes and again give them a few seconds to rest.

Exercise 2

Same as exercise one but instead of looking left and right look up and down.

Exercise 3

Extend your right arm in front of yourself and in a horizontal position. Extend your thumb so that you are looking at the thumbnail. Focus your eyes on the tip of your thumb. Try not to blink. Slowly start to move your hand towards your nose. Keep focusing on the same spot as you are doing that. When the finger touches the tip of your nose hold it there for one or more seconds and then slowly return your hand to the starting position still keeping the same point in focus. At the end of the exercise blink a few times and relax.

Exercise 4

When you first begin doing eye exercises it is wise to avoid over-stressing your muscles. In that context one should begin by avoiding the full range of motion in any eye exercise. This principle is particularly true for this exercise in which you roll your eyes. To do this exercise start by rolling your eyes in small circles. As you feel your way through the exercise increase the size of the circles in which you roll your eyes until you reach your maximum. Do 5-10 rolls clockwise. Relax your eyes by closing them for a few seconds. Repeat the same number of rolls counterclockwise.

Exercise 5

Blink rapidly. Repeat the exercise 10 - 20 times. Close your eyes and lightly massage them with the tips of your fingers. Before doing that rub your fingers together until they are warm.

Exercise 6

This exercise is performed standing up and in front of a sink. First, fill a large bowl with clean water and place it in the sink. Then fill your mouth with clean water. Bend forward keeping your eyes wide open and your mouth closed. Inhale through your nose, then exhale fully through your nose. Put your hands together so that your palms touch each other. Using your hands splash some water into your open eyes trying not to blink. It will take a few days until you will learn how to correctly perform this exercise. Splash water in your eyes until the water in your mouth becomes warm. This will take approximately 10 - 20 splashes. Spit out the water from your mouth, dry your face with a towel and lightly massage your closed eyes.

Therapeutic Effects

The cold water in your mouth stimulates blood flow in the area of the face, nose and eyes; and improves your vision. Rinsing your eyes with water acts as a massage. It has a good effect on the muscles of the eye and on circulation, and tones the nerve endings in the eyes. *The exercises for eyes described in this book strengthen the eye muscles, improve circulation and (if performed regularly) can actually improve vision for some people, depending on personal circumstances.*

Suggestions on Maintaining Your Vision

To make sure that eye exercises yield better results it is important to make vision hygiene a part of your daily life.

1. Don't read or write too closely to the text. Its best to keep the text at a distance of your half stretched arm. Lighting should be bright enough without the light heating the eyes directly.
2. During long and strenuous eye work give yourself a break for 3 - 5 minutes every 20-60 minutes. During that time it good to look at a pretty landscape at a distance or massage your eyes.
3. When watching television do so from a distance of about six times the width of the TV screen. There should additional lighting with light not heating the screen or your eyes directly.
4. It is recommended to look at a distance on trees, flowers, water, sky, and clouds.

It not only gives rest to the eyes but also calms down nervous system, improves mood and takes your mind off negative thoughts and emotions.

Lyme-My Life was over

My husband brought me to Dr. Koyfman in a wheelchair. I had Lyme disease which progressed into severe MS and other illnesses. I could not function. My whole body was in pain. I could not even take a shower on my own. After speaking to Dr. Koyfman, we realized how knowledgeable he is and decided to give it a shot.

After only a few of his cleansing procedures I was a different person. Every day I was getting stronger and stronger. I started slowly, but got all of my body functions back. Now a couple of years later, I am still amazed with Dr. Koyfman's abilities. I feel better than I felt even before I got ill. My muscles do not hurt. I am full of energy. My family is amazed that I have more energy than all of them together. Even my hair and teeth look better than ever. Thanks to Dr. Koyfman I have a new life style, eating habits, and the whole perspective of life. I am a happy mom and wife and tend to stay that way forever.

I have referred many people with these horrible disease to Dr. Koyfman and all of them had great success. He doesn't want to admit it, but we all think it might just be the cure!

Carol G., Age 34

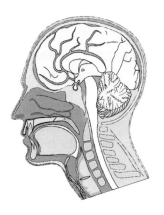

Thyroid Gland

The Role of the Thyroid Glands

The thyroid gland is found at the base of the neck, toward the front. It is composed of two lobes, one on each side of the windpipe. **The thyroid is responsible for regulating the metabolism,** the term used to describe the many processes that take place in the body.

The thyroid gland is part of the endocrine system. This system regulates the body's production and use of hormones. Hormones control virtually every fundamental human function, including growth and development, maturation, reproduction and most of human behavior. **The thyroid gland is a fortress to protect the system from invasion by many diseases.**

Sabotaging the Thyroid Glands

If your thyroid gland is sluggish, you may experience physical and mental sluggishness, problems losing weight, decreased body temperature, puffiness in the hands and face, goiter, and an enlarged thyroid gland. When your thyroid is overactive, you may experience extreme nervousness, weight loss or difficulty gaining weight, rapid pulse, bulging eyes and heart failure.

White refined sugar has an adverse effect on the thyroid gland. Too much sugar is one of the causes of osteoporosis. You can take large amount of calcium and you won't get much benefit from it without reducing your intake of sugar.

Emotional stress can have a powerfully adverse effect on the thyroid.

Checking the Thyroid Glands Yourself

If you suspect that your thyroid gland is not functioning properly you can easily test it yourself without the need of going to a doctor. All you have to do is to place a thermometer on your night stand or any other place where you can easily reach it from your bed. Do this before going to bed. When you awaken after a full night's sleep, reach for the thermometer and take your temperature. This should be done as the absolutely first thing you do upon waking, before you make any other movements. If you temperature is normal, then your thyroid glands are in good shape. If the temperature is elevated, then the functions of the thyroid glands are elevated. If the temperature is below normal, then the functions of thyroid gland are decreased. In serious cases it is necessary to have professional testing done.

Causes of Poor Thyroid Gland Functioning

Disruption in the work of the thyroid glands can be due to:

1. Your blood being polluted with toxins and heavy metals which block gland ducts and membranes,
2. Poor blood circulation (which results from the blockages described above),
3. Lack of proper exercising which slows blood circulation,
4. Tension remaining in glands and muscles by stress,
5. Insufficient nutrition due to incorrect diet and presence of parasites.

Therefore, it becomes apparent that to regain normal functioning of these glands, it is important to eliminate all of the causes described above.

Pollution of the blood is dealt with by cleansing the large intestine, liver and lymph glands.

Reestablishing the normal circulation of blood is done by exercises, massage, sauna, and warm baths.

Dealing with tension in organs is discussed below.

Methods of Cleansing and Improving the Health of the Thyroid Glands

Physical Techniques for increasing blood circulation and cleansing the thyroid gland include:

1. Exercises for the neck are discussed in my book *Unique Method of Colon Rejuvenation.*

2. Shoulder Stand - See a good book on yoga. Exercise 2 brings a lot of blood which concentrates in the thyroid gland, enriching it with essential nutrients while soaking and softening the waste in the gland. Exercises 3 and 4, when done after this one, stretch the neck and thyroid gland, making its ducts more open and flexible and flushing the toxins away from it.

3. Cobra pose - See a good book on yoga.

4. Fish pose - See a good book on yoga.

5. Take a piece of clean cloth, drop 3-7 drops of iodine on it, and gently massage the area of the thyroid gland. Do this massage 2 times per day for 2-3 minutes.

6. Finger massage of the tongue, described in the chapter entitled, "Tongue." This massage doesn't just cleanse the tongue but it has many additional wonderful benefits. It also helps to cleanse the thyroid glands. You can do this procedure every day, since it takes hardly any time.

7. Juice from the black radish cleanses the thyroid gland and improves its function. In my center, I've seen many cases of an improving thyroid gland after using black radish juice. These were proven not only by feeling better and more healthy, but also by medical tests. In nature, the black radish is available in late fall; therefore, it has the largest effect when used in fall, winter, or early spring. **Recipe:** Clean the radishes very carefully. If you find organic radishes, you may use them without peeling. Make 2-3 quarts of juice, put in a glass jar, cover, and put in the refrigerator. Drink 2-3 times per day, 30 minutes before a meal beginning with 1 teaspoon and gradually increasing to 2-3 tablespoons and more. Repeat the procedure 1-2 times per year.

Relieving tensions in organs caused by stress can be achieved through breathing exercises, plus relaxation, meditation and cleansing procedures. Cleansing the main excretory channels opens the door to eliminate physical and emotional toxins from other organs, including the thyroid glands.

Improvement of nutrition in the body is done by clearing up digestion problems through stomach cleansing, small intestine and liver cleansing, removal of parasites, followed by a healthy diet and supplements.

The functions of the thyroid glands are positively affected by being on or near the ocean and eating seafood products rich in iodine. These foods include kelp, seaweed, and fish.

Some vegetables good for thyroid gland health are: radishes, watercress, collards and other leafy greens, squash, carrots, and broccoli. Some grain products good for thyroid gland health are: corn, wheat and millet.

Also good are vitamins A, B6 and E and minerals zinc and copper.

The Next Book

The abdominal area is the kitchen of our bodies. How well or poorly this kitchen functions depends on whether we feed our system with nutrients or poison our system with toxicity. If your abdominal kitchen produces nutrients, you are getting health; if your kitchen produces poison, you are getting disease.

How can you help your abdominal organs to become more healthy and free of toxins and sustain the health of your entire body? You will find the answers in the pages of the *Healing through Cleansing, Book 3.*

This book also contains information on other important cleansings which may prevent disease or even help to heal in the following organs and systems:

*   How to Improve and Stretch the Immune System with:
    *   Cleansing of Lymphatic Fluid and Lymph Nodes.
    *   Parasite Cleansing with Food and Herbs.
    *   Cleansing from Heavy Metals.
    *   Cleansing from Negative Emotions.
    *   Cleansing the Sexual Organs to Help Healing and Prevention of Disease in the Reproductive Organs.
    *   Ten Simple Techniques to Cleanse Blood Vessels.
    *   Simple Way to Help to Heal Hemorrhoids.
    *   Cleansing the Joints and Spine.
    *   And More . . .

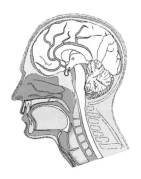

Testimonials

"My Allergies Have Gotten Better"

I followed Dr. Koyfman's preventive treatment procedures for three to four months. Now I feel so much better, and my allergies have gotten better. Dr. Koyfman helped me coordinate my diet. He knows what he is doing, and most important of all he lives what he teaches. For him it's not just a business, it is lifestyle.

—Alla Spivak

"I Have *Much* More Energy"

I really like coming here because, first of all, it's really fun. I enjoy the conversation and the laughter and the not taking everything so seriously. Also, I learn a lot; I can ask all the questions I want. It's nice to learn Russian, too.

The main thing I've noticed since coming here is that I have *much* more energy. Also, my eyes definitely look better, and

I've lost weight. I used to be very lethargic in the mornings and now I actually get up earlier and with more energy. I've learned a lot and feel much better and really want to stay young because I met the man of my dreams and he's ten years younger.

Once you get over the uncomfortableness/awkwardness of the first colonic, it becomes much easier and quite interesting to see what comes out.

I recommend not lying about what you eat because Yakov "knows when you've been bad or good, so be good for goodness' sake."

—Claire Vohman

"Happier, Healthier, and Thinner"

Healing of the body can never occur without cleansing . . . especially the digestive tract.

Atlanta is very fortunate that Russian Naturopath, Yakov Koyfman, has decided to settle in our city.

A naturopath uses only natural methods to cure disorders. Dr. Koyfman spent over 24 years learning techniques of natural healing in Russia, China, and Europe. Along with a very loving and caring staff, Dr. Koyfman can guide you through the process of cleansing the liver, gall bladder, colon, small intestines, and stomach. Everyone I know who has gone to him feels happier, healthier, and thinner, and is clearly much more bright and energetic.

—Donna Gates
Author of the book, *The Body Ecology Diet*

"Bronchitis for Over Ten Years"

I have suffered from bronchitis and respiratory problems for over ten years. I was sick with bronchial infections for several weeks at least twice every year. Medical doctors repeatedly told me that I had chronic bronchitis, and they treated the condition with antibiotics. However, my immune system became weakened, and I was constantly sick with colds and laryngitis. It appeared as though the antibiotics had become somewhat ineffective. As the bronchial condition worsened, I was diagnosed as having asthma.

After suffering from asthma for almost a year with my doctor treating the disease with steroid pills and several types of nasal and oral inhalers, my condition had grown progressively worse. I became weakened from coughing, wheezing, and choking for air. I would awaken from my sleep coughing and choking during the night. I could hardly climb a flight of stairs without becoming short of breath, weak, and tired. I felt helpless and honestly thought that I was going to die from this disease.

It was absolutely a providence that my daughter worked for a naturopathic doctor during this time. My daughter advised me to see this doctor. Although I was not quite familiar with natural healing then, I knew that I desperately needed help and went to see the doctor. After consulting with me the doctor said, "You are full of toxins. Your eyes are puffed. Your face is swollen. Your joints are stiff and swollen. And you are bloated. You need to see Dr. Koyfman." The doctor's nurse called Dr. Koyfman's office and made an appointment for me. I saw him that very afternoon.

The year was 1999. It was the week before Christmas when Dr. Koyfman began treating me. After just a few treatments of colonics I began to breathe better and feel stronger. Dr. Koyfman developed a treatment plan to fit my need and care, and I began the program with focus and discipline. Now almost a year later, I am honored to testify to the world and say that I no longer take medications for asthma and palpitations. My blood pressure and cholesterol results are normal. I have lost 30 pounds. I am lean, stronger, and full of energy, but most of all I am well and healthy.

Dr. Koyfman is an excellent Naturopathic Doctor and teacher. In my opinion, he is one of the best doctors in his business. His ultimate objective is to restore patients' wellness. Dr. Koyfman taught me how to take better care of myself. For example, I learned the value of exercise, how to adjust to a healthy lifestyle, and most of all the wholeness of food. Dr. Koyfman and his staff care about their patients and provide their patients with excellent service. I am grateful to Dr. Koyfman for my wellness and my quality of life. I feel that God has healed me through Dr. Koyfman's hands. I am thankful to Mrs. Koyfman for her support and excellent care, and to Alex for his kindness and good cheer during the difficult times.

- Joyce Martin

My Dear Koyfman Folks -

Just wanted to let you know I've completed my 4th Liver Cleanse. It's been an amazing experience.

You people working at Dr Koyfman's office are wonderful, kind, considerate and did your best to answer questions. I never had to wait for my appointment. If anything, you would take me early. This took the stress off of having to wait that normally comes with going to a Dr.'s office.

I no longer have acid reflux, and I have lost 30 lbs. I started at 154 and am happy to say I now weigh 124. I've learned to appreciate my body and my body's needs. Dr Koyfman is so knowledgeable about our bodies and what it needs to run efficiently without all the medications so easily passed out in the "medical world". I really mistreated myself eating the way I did, and this resulted in feeling tired most of the time. I've learned to eat properly with correct food combinations and now I have so much more energy.

I do believe cleansing our bodies to get rid of toxins is an important part of our health. I'm 52 years old and I still have a lot of living to do. I want to feel well doing it, and I sure don't want to be left behind while the rest of my family and friends are have a good time. I'll continue on a maintenance program to keep this body I live in well tuned.

Olga, thank you for being such a sweetie and making my colonics enjoyable. We had some fun conversations. I wish you joy and happiness always.

Helen and Mrs. Koyfman. Thank you for sharing your knowledge with me.

Dr. Koyfman, you are a gifted man and thank you for pursuing your career and sharing all you've learned with so many people thru the years. God bless you, your family and the ones working at your Clinic.

I'll be seeing you again.

-- Diane

Shearer--

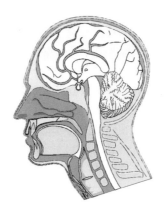

About our Cleansing Center

Philosophy and Services

The Immune System and Toxicity

Living today is hard on the body! Environmental poisons, food additives, stresses at home and at work, plus a wide diversity of other stresses come together to overload the body's resources. Resulting tensions, wastes, parasites, and many illnesses which thrive in such conditions produce poisons throughout the body. These are the poisons that weaken the body on its way to the grave.

God created within the body its own cleansing organs and systems (colon, kidneys, skin, lungs, lymph) which work to eradicate the incoming toxins. This system is both brilliant and powerful. To ignore it is to short circuit the wisest physician you can ever have working for you.

However, this system is not perfect. Bringing the power of the mind to work with this system can increase its effectiveness immensely. This is done when the mind realizes the wonderful array of cleansing techniques available to the body. It also happens when good nutritional practices are implemented.

There is another consideration. Each person's body has different strengths and weaknesses. For example, one person's liver is powerful while another's is not. Conversely, the person with a weaker liver has a stronger colon. The permutations on this are endless, and are due to genetic makeup, lifestyle and personal history. Because of this tremendous individuality in strengths and weaknesses, professionals trained in natural health care and cleansing are a powerful ally and weapon in the fight for optimal health.

Since the body gradually accumulates more and more stored toxins, which continue to poison their host, the immune system, driven to neutralize the effects of the stored poisons, becomes overworked and weakened.

As life goes on, the toxins accumulate to the extent that they create blockages in one or several vital channels such as arteries and other blood vessels, liver ducts, kidneys, breathing passages, or the digestive tract. These blockages have become the major causes of death in today's world.

Good diet, proper exercise, and healthy lifestyle can reduce incoming toxins and increase outgoing toxins, but they cannot stop the accumulation. Toxins do continue to enter and accumulate, coming as they do, not only from food, but also from environmental and other sources beyond our control and common to our daily lives.

One way to reduce the toxicity in the body to a level that is not dangerous, and then to maintain this level, is to use cleansing procedures.

What Are Cleansing Procedures?

Cleansing procedures are specifically designed to help the body eliminate accumulated waste and poison from internal organs, vital channels, and cells. Any treatment of illness will not yield long-term health improvement if these toxins are not eliminated from the body. Cleansing procedures do this work quickly and effectively.

Cleansing procedures in our Center use only natural means and methods. Clean water, herbs, fresh juices, massage of internal organs, heat, and special solutions help to dissolve the wastes and poisons stored in the various organs. Our Center's state-of-the-art cleansing and massage equipment serves to protect and enhance the natural processes of the body. This includes equipment to perform lymph drainage, lymph node cleansing, sinus cleansing, heavy metals elimination, and an infrared sauna.

List of Cleansing Procedures Available in Our Center

- Cleansing the Whole Digestive System
- Stomach Cleansing
- Pancreas Cleansing
- Liver Cleansing
- Gallbladder Cleansing
- Small Intestine Cleansing
- Colon Cleansing
- Joint Cleansing
- Kidney Cleansing
- Lung Cleansing
- Sinus Cleansing
- Infrared Sauna Cleansing
- Whole Body Cleansing Massage
- Internal Organ Massage
- *Cleansing to Improve the Immune System*
- Parasite Cleansing
- Heavy Metals Cleansing
- Cleansing from Negative Emotions
- Lymph Cleansing and Lymph Drainage
- Cell Cleansing
- Thyroid Cleansing Program
- Prostate Cleansing Program
- Weight Loss Cleansing Program

More detailed information about these services and procedures can be found at our website www.koyfmancenter.com, in pamphlets available in our office, and in my book, *Eight Steps to Perfect Health.*

Symptoms of High Level Toxicity

✓   Constipation
✓   Gas
✓   Bloating
✓   Liver Problems
✓   Gall Bladder Stones
✓   Pancreas Problems
✓   Parasites
✓   Hemorrhoids
✓   Skin Problems
✓   Allergies
✓   Asthma
✓   High Cholesterol
✓   Sinus Problems
✓   Joint Pain/ Back Pain
✓   High Blood Pressure
✓   Tiredness/ Fatigue
✓   Insomnia
✓   Nervousness
✓   Obesity

How Soon Can a Person Feel Better with These Procedures?

Everything is individualized. One person may find some improvement after the first procedure. In other cases, it takes more time. One thing that anyone and everyone agrees on is that the removal of poisons, toxins, and wastes from the body will improve one's health.

What Procedures Does a Person Need?

The beginning of any cleansing program requires colon cleansing, as consideration of this picture will illustrate.

What's Wrong With This Picture?

The colon depicted here is suffering from being stuffed with undigested food, toxic mucus, fermenting wastes, putrefied feces, and gas that has a similar toxic chemical composition.

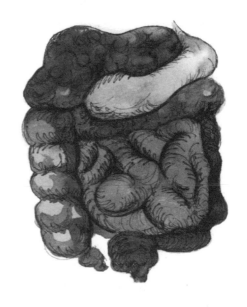

A colon thus *expanded* with old fecal matter, gas, and new food puts pressure on neighboring organs. This pressure can hinder and sometimes seriously block the circulation of fluids in, to and around these organs. This interferes with the natural removal of wastes, and the delivery of oxygen and nutrients.

Chemically, such a wretched colon has the necessary environmental (anaerobic) conditions for starting and supporting all kinds of unwanted biological organisms, such as parasites, worms, viruses, and bacteria. Toxins stuck to the colon wall are absorbed through the colon walls, and spread to other organs and systems all over the body. Once in their new home or repository they form either toxic mucous or crystals the size of sand or small stones. These then become problems that poison and weaken the system further.

This same kind of process has been found operating in the arteries, veins, and other passages throughout the body. Plaque building up on the walls of blood vessels and arteries is one of the more famous examples of this basic process. This makes the heart's work more difficult and translates to feelings of tiredness and fatigue.

For prevention, our Center recommends cleansing of the large intestine or colon, followed by a systematic cleansing of the major organs. Parasite cleansing would complete the basic program. Once the vast majority of the body's organs are cleansed, a maintenance program would be part of the healthy lifestyle.

To solve a specific health problem, we can tailor an individualized program which will include cleansing procedures (such as Stomach Cleansing, Cleansing the Whole Digestive System, Small Intestine Cleansing, Liver Cleansing, etc.), diet, exercise, and other components necessary to creating a healthy lifestyle. The more serious the problem, the more time is required.

Proof of the benefit of the cleansing procedures may be seen after the first to fifth cleansing procedures. You will begin to feel better and have more energy. Your immune system will become stronger. Gradually the problem will become less, and for many people it will disappear.

In our Center the client also receives education in right eating, healthy recipes, cleansing exercises, and the healthy lifestyle.

Dr. Yakov Koyfman, Naturopathic Doctor

As early as 1976, Dr. Koyfman was interested in alternative medicine in Ukraine, Russia. His first experiments were on himself, as he helped his own sinus and digestive problems, back pain, and colds. Then he did extensive study and self-research under famous doctors from India, Russia, and Japan. He studied nutrition, dietology, and fasting therapy in Russia. He is certified by the American (and Georgia State) Naturopathic Medical Association. He is certified also by the International Association for Colon HydroTherapy (I.-A.C.T.). He holds a diploma as a European and Oriental Massage Therapist (First Degree), and a diploma from the National Board of Naturopathic Examiners. His system combines experience, knowledge, and techniques from the East and from the West.

In 1994, Dr. Koyfman founded his Center in America, and has helped thousands of people since then. People come for help from not only Atlanta, but also from other states and countries including Florida, Washington, and New York, Canada, Germany, Israel, and Russia.

Dr. Koyfman has authored many articles and books where he describes his health philosophy. You can order these books from the Center, or buy them in some near by health food stores.

Awaken! It is not Too Late... Yet

Two processes of destruction and rehabilitation lead the fight in the human body from the moment of birth and to the end of the life. When we are young, the rehabilitation process is dominating where as process of destruction is still weak and not as significant. However, when we reach approximately thirty years of age (or even sooner) the destruction process grows stronger making the rehabilitation process weaker.

So what exactly is being destructed in the human body?

The cells of the body become clogged and overfilled with toxicity, loose their elasticity and begin to age. Skin and tissue stretch and hang. Joint glands clog-up and produce less lubrication causing joint bones to rub against each other. Gradually joints rub off and coverup with salt crystals and uric acid. Polluted large intestine (colon) contaminates blood, blood vessels and lymph - slowing down circulation. The heart exhausts by trying to overcome the pressure in the colon and by pushing the blood through clogged-up vessels, and finally wears off. The energy drops drastically. Glands of internal secretion also become clogged. Lowers production and secretion of vital hormones. Slowly, but surely all organs and systems become congested and polluted, which significantly lowers their functioning. The body accumulates and produces more and more toxicity, and less nutrients to feed the immune system. The protection system weakens. Unfriendly bacteria, infection and other parasites meet less and less resistance from the immune system and reproduce easily. These creatures eat our nutrients, organs and muscles. They eat us alive! The body's resistance to destruction lowers rapidly and our unthoughtful actions speed up the process even more. The border line becomes closer and closer.

So how can you slow down that persistent stream of time? That process of destruction?

In my books Healing Through Cleansing volumes 1-4, find answers on how to rid of many illnesses and stay healthy and young until a 100 and beyond.

Unique Method of Colon Rejuvenation, 95 pages; $12.

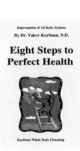

Our bodies need constant help eliminating toxic substances which enter the system every day. Daily practice of the rising and restroom exercises described in this book strengthens colon muscles so that, with time, elimination will accompany each meal and eject more toxins than are retained. Also included are principles and recipes for healthy eating, raw meals, and safe cooking technology.

Eight Steps to Total Body Cleansing and Perfect Health, 214 pages; $20.

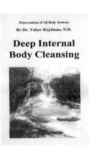

You will find here how to prepare for cleansing and what to expect during Deep Internal Body Cleansing. You will want to know what to do if you feel any discomfort during the cleansing. This book explains how we perform Deep Internal Body Cleansing at the Center. Also, you will discover here what to eat after the cleansing in order to maintain your success and your new lifestyle.

Deep Internal Body Cleansing, 172 pages. $15 plus shipping and handling.

If you search for healing and real health, then here you will find answers to your questions Here is information about toxicity and the immune system, healthy eating and eliminating parasites. Here are answers to help you resist hurtful cravings and negative emotions. You really can get health and gain energy through cleansing your body.

Healing Through Cleansing - Book 1, 114 pages; $12.

Every day, toxic substances enter our bodies from the various chemical and biological contaminants in our environment. Additionally, toxins form within us due to poor dietary habits, stress, aging, and harmful bacteria that populate our bodies. Our excretory organs can't cope with such a large amount of work and need constant, conscious support. How can you help your main excretory organs become free of toxins, bacteria, and infections? You will find the answers in the pages of this and subsequent books in this Koyfman Series.

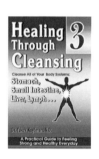

Healing Through Cleansing - Book 3, 120 pages; $12.

The abdominal area is the kitchen of our bodies. How well or poorly this kitchen functions depends on whether we feed our system with nutrients or poison our system with toxicity. If your abdominal kitchen produces nutrients, you are getting health; if your kitchen produces poison, you are getting disease. How can you help your abdominal organs to become more healthy and free of toxins and to sustain the health of your entire body? You will find the answers in the pages of this book.

Healing Through Cleansing Diet - Book 4, 116 pages; $12.

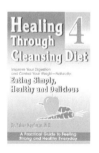

"To get the best results in the healing process, it is not enough to find a skilled teacher who can guide you along the path. It is also very important that the student be open-minded to new information and ready to work," says Dr. Yakov Koyfman, N.D. A healthy diet gives to the system not only nutrients but also help to clean and heal the body. To make your diet healthy, you need to learn the things in this book.